The Revolution of Naturopathic Medicine
Remaining True to Our Philosophy

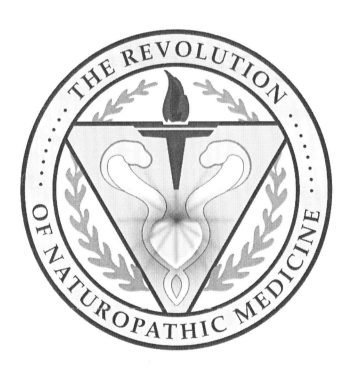

Moshe Daniel Block, ND, HMC

Collective Co-op Publishing
Montreal, Quebec
Canada
publishing@collectivecoop.com

2nd Edition. ISBN 0-9731406-2-3

Contents

Naturopathic Physician's Oath

I dedicate myself to the service of humanity as a practitioner of the art and science of Naturopathic medicine.

I will honor my teachers and all who have preserved and developed this knowledge and dedicate myself to supporting the growth and evolution of Naturopathic medicine. I will endeavor to continually improve my abilities as a healer through study, reflection, and genuine concern for humanity. I will impart knowledge of the advanced healing arts to dedicated colleagues and students.

Through precept, lecture, and example, I will assist and encourage others to strengthen their health, reduce risks for disease, and preserve the health of our planet for ourselves, our families, and future generations.

According to my best ability and judgment, I will use methods of treatment which follow the principles of Naturopathic medicine:

First of all, to do no harm.
To act in cooperation with the Healing Power of Nature.
To address the fundamental causes of disease.
To heal the whole person through individualized treatment.
To teach the principles of healthy living and preventive medicine.

I will conduct my life and the practice of Naturopathic health care with vigilance, integrity, and freedom from prejudice. I will abstain from voluntary acts of injustice and corruption. I will keep confidential whatever I am privileged to witness, whether professionally or privately, that should not be divulged.

With my whole heart, before this gathering of witnesses, as a Doctor of Naturopathic Medicine, I pledge to remain true to this oath.

Foreword

Naturopathy, which began as a reform movement, is now itself in need of reform. It is probably already too late to make such pronouncements as, "Naturopathy stands at a crossroads," or, "Naturopathy is facing an identity crisis." In embracing so-called "Evidence-based Medicine" (EBM), naturopathy has already, consciously or unconsciously, embarked on a new path and chosen a new identity that is in fundamental contradiction to and a negation of its historical roots and the vision of such founding figures as Benedict Lust and Henry Lindlahr.

EBM is a product of the mechanistic world-view. The most basic tenet of this world-view is that the human sense faculties and mind are inherently faulty and subjective, and the claims of all empirical traditions such as naturopathy must be dismissed until each, one-by-one, can be demonstrated by "valid research" as "hard facts." In this view, only phenomena that can be measured with the so-called "objective" instruments of science are considered as real. Therefore, all ancient medical traditions must be considered as superstitions, as such basic concepts as Qi (Chinese medicine), prana (Ayurvedic medicine) and vital force (naturopathic and homeopathic medicines), among many others, cannot be measured and verified by external experiments and instruments. They can only be experienced, and experience is denied as a source of valid information.

Many critics and philosophers of science since the time of Goethe have pointed out the numerous flaws inherent in the mechanistic world-view and the scientific method. Although this is not the forum to enumerate these criticisms, it is worth noting here that the so-called "objective realm," on which its judgments about what is real and not real hinges, is itself a product of the subjective mind, and therefore must also be subjective. It has not been discovered, but rather invented. The holistic scientist and poet Goethe demonstrated that mechanism, materialism, reductionism or whatever name we choose is itself a system of belief rather than a set of facts. Its hallowed scientific method, revered and unquestioned for its success in producing the amazing advances we see in technology, produces not facts but hypotheses. If, as the critic and philosopher of science Karl Popper has pointed out, "Science is the set of hypotheses not yet falsified," then the evidence generated by EBM using the scientific method need not be regarded as real or of special merit. It is ephemeral, and as experience repeatedly demonstrates, bound one day to be discarded.

In his 1923 classic, *Philosophy of Natural Therapeutics*, Lindlahr specifically points (p. 16) to another way of knowing. He writes, "the simple pioneers of Nature Cure...refused to be blinded or confused by the conflicting theories of books and authorities," but rather that they, "applied common sense reasoning," and, "went for inspiration to field and forest," while studying, "the whole and not only the parts, causes as well as effects and symptoms." This is the way of holism, contemplation of nature in "field and forest," with the understanding common to Chinese and Ayurvedic medicines that the external and internal environments of humans are one and the same. This is a recognition of the essential "Oneness" implied in the word universe. In this view, human intelligence and the senses which inform it, although indeed prone to error, are formed of the Supreme Intelligence, and can therefore be refined to know and apprehend truth directly without the intervention of artificial experiments based on speculative theories. Furthermore, those who depend on such theories at the expense of their "common sense reasoning" wind up "blinded or confused."

The naturopathy of Lust, Lindlahr and others represented a movement toward a vitalistic and holistic science of western medicine that can perhaps stand one day with Chinese and India=s Ayurvedic Medicines as one of the great comprehensive systems of natural healing. Lindlahr pointedly denounces what he calls the materialistic world view as absurd (pp. 23–4), and proposes rather that there is a vital force, a "supreme intelligence and Power acting in and through every atom, molecule and cell in the human body." Matter, rather than being the source of life through its random and mechanical operations, is "but an expression of the Life Force, itself a manifestation of the great Creative Intelligence." In this view, irreconcilable with mechanism and EBM, the universe is a product of Consciousness, and "All things in nature, from a fleeting thought or emotion to the hardest piece of diamond or platinum, are modes of motion or vibration," and "If [the] supreme Intelligence should withdraw its creative energy…the entire material universe would disappear in the flash of a moment." That is to say, all things continuously flow from the One.

In his 1902 publication, The Naturopathic and Herald of Health, Benedict Lust described naturopathy as, "the reconciling, harmonizing and unifying of nature, humanity and God," and spoke of the "surpassing achievement of our world-wide purpose." Lindlahr (p15) saw it as, "a complete revolution in the art and science of living. It is the practical realization and application of all that is good in natural science, philosophy and religion." Surely these are grand visions of a holistic art and science of life and medicine. The embrace of EBM and the reductionistic approach to science by the profession effectively ends any possibility other than becoming an adjunct to the dominant system already in place. While this may seem desirable as offering a niche within the corporate Health Care Industry to our field, it abolishes the identity, tradition and promise of the profession. Although we cannot enter into a suitable discussion of the much-abused term "holistic" in this space, suffice it to say that the reductionistic method of EBM must separate and break down in order to isolate phenomena in its search for facts. This is a violation of the basic holistic tenet that phenomena can only be understood in the context of their environment, and that any attempt to artificially isolate any phenomenon must of necessity change that phenomenon. I do not mean to imply here that naturopaths should discard all results brought to light by the laser beam of reductionistic science, but rather that those results must be illuminated in the sunshine of holism in order to be properly understood. I certainly do mean, however, that we cannot at once be holistic and reductionistic, and that if we are to consider ourselves to be truly scientific and holistic, we must work to produce a rigorous, clear and comprehensive holistic science of medicine that builds on the ancient traditions handed to us.

If naturopathy is to have any future other than that of generic complementary alternative medicine, it must reform. Our forebears in this profession provided us with a foundation of holism and vitalism on which to build. The *vis medicatrix naturae* is eternal and as strong as ever, and will be there for us when we are ready to again join forces with it. In this book, Daniel Block raises an impassioned voice imploring us to do just that. He offers us an updated view of the traditional naturopathic philosophy that speaks to our time, and a critique of our educational system that should be considered by everyone interested in the direction and future of our profession. Furthermore, he encourages us to face and lay aside the fear and insecurity that drive the profession toward a need for acceptance and credibility from mainstream medicine. Our forebears saw clearly that the mechanist philosophy is itself an illness, a delusion. How can we be part of healing if we ourselves have the disease?

George Savastio, ND

Introduction

NATUROPATHIC MEDICINE faces a great challenge, a challenge faced by every profession that fails to follow the principles and philosophy upon which it was founded. Improving this situation will require the determination and commitment from the students and practitioners of naturopathic medicine. The dilemma we face within our profession is the challenge of identity: can we be successful remaining true to our identity by practicing our medicine hand in hand with our philosophy, or must we seek recognition and credibility by emulating the way of established medicine?

The answer to this question is very simple: Naturopathic medicine will bring better health to the world and gain recognition from the public and the medical establishment when our medicine is practiced as it was conceived—in harmony with Nature and with the principles of our philosophy. Any attempts to gain recognition by emulating the ways of other medicines can only weaken our profession.

This book is a discussion of how to remain true to our philosophy and why remaining true to our philosophy is absolutely essential at this time. This book will clarify each of the principles of our philosophy and explain how one can employ these principles to heal people. This book dispels much of the fear and doubt that arise when one practices whole person medicine, walking a path that is not yet fully accepted or established in society. In fact, this book encourages the student and doctor of naturopathy to facilitate the switch in medicine from the allopathic paradigm to the healing paradigm, in harmony with our philosophy. All the discussions within these pages encourage the practice of the pure form of our medicine and the letting go of ways that have been adopted from other medicines.

There is a pure form of practicing Naturopathy that aligns it with the healing power of Nature (Vis Medicatrix Naturae—aka

1

The Vis) and provides the longest lasting and deepest influence on a person's health and well-being. The pure form also helps patients and doctors understand that we all have the power over, and responsibility for, our own health. Whole person naturopathic medicine ensures that a doctor understands how to act in harmony with Nature without claiming all responsibility for people's health, and it does not attempt to manipulate the symptoms of disease to create the false appearance of health. Having a basis in the true form of naturopathy gives one a working foundation for dealing with all expressions of illness.

Not everyone agrees with the definition of naturopathic medicine. I understand that there are many different ways of practicing. What I hope to establish is the understanding that the people we treat are best served when we practice in harmony with our philosophy. That philosophy is not my opinion; rather, it is something that has existed for many years. Even though the *interpretation* of the philosophy is left up to each person, when we work in harmony with Nature, even in the myriad ways of expressing our medicine, there is a commonality because *we share the way of the healing paradigm.* Thus the way of our philosophy, which is the way of naturopathic medicine, is not defined by a rigid set of rules that all must adhere to, but rather is governed by the healing power of Nature itself that all can recognize. So let this book be an inspiration for those practitioners and students already embracing our philosophy and let them find confirmation in the expression of naturopathic philosophy on these pages. Let this book also be an encouragement for those who do not work closely with our philosophy to gain some insight into the essence of naturopathic medicine and to find reasons for adopting as much of the philosophy as they feel comfortable with.

When we graduate, the first line of our oath includes the following words: "I dedicate myself to the service of humanity as a practitioner of the art and science of naturopathic medicine." We owe it not only to ourselves to be true to our philosophy at every phase of the education process and out in the field, but we owe it to all people on this planet who are seeking answers to the deeper questions of their health and well-being.

Although our medicine has existed for thousands of years, it is emerging again today on the cutting edge of the healing world. Today's diseases call for deeper solutions to chronic problems that cannot be solved solely on the physical dimension. The number of people embracing alternative medicines canopied beneath the healing paradigm grows every day. People yearn for us to carry our medicine forward in the way in which it was conceived, rather than emulate a medicine that can no longer provide them with solutions to many manifestations of disease.

Naturopathic medicine is a gift to the world because it offers solutions to the rising costs of healthcare by using treatments that are relatively inexpensive. It also solves the problem of iatrogenesis in medicine since practicing whole person naturopathy is completely gentle, thereby fulfilling the principle; "Do no harm." One of the greatest gifts that comes from naturopathic medicine arises from doctors fulfilling their role as teacher, helping people understand the connection between their minds—their life choices and way of thinking—their bodies, and their overall health. Naturopathic medicine does not simply give people a fish for a day, but it teaches them how to fish for themselves, giving them tools to live in happier and more holistic lives.

The born naturopath is attracted to this profession because he/she recognizes it to be a medicine of healing. The wish to learn how to embody our philosophy comes from the person's heart and soul, which is the heart and soul of a healer, a doctor of Nature. Such a person also understands the great necessity in his/her own inner work and transformation in order to comprehend the healing process as a whole and the way it functions in others. Therefore, this book suggests placing a great emphasis on Hippocrates' famous statement, "Physician, Heal Thyself!" in the curriculum by offering many courses that would involve the inner work of self-healing and transformation. The blind cannot lead the blind, nor can the sick heal the sick. This is one of the necessary steps in the right direction to help doctors graduate as more effective tools in the proper care of their patients.

This book also examines the education, the clinic, and the practice of naturopathic medicine to see that those parts are brought into harmony with the pure form of our medicine. It is especially important that the education of naturopathic medicine be aligned with the roots of naturopathic medicine from the very beginning of the program until the day we graduate. This book critiques the current model of naturopathic medical education and gives suggestions for change. It takes a close look at such elements as the screening process, the courses of the curriculum, the clinic, and the licensing exams, and discusses how all can be aligned with the essence of our medicine to fulfill the purpose of creating effective, safe, and confident naturopaths highly skilled in the use of various modalities.

As it now stands, there are elements of naturopathic medicinal education not very well aligned with the principles of our medicine. Whatever the reasons, these elements are dividing our profession between the allopathic and naturopathic way. Anything so divided cannot carry out its purpose. Our graduates are therefore not fully prepared in either the allopathic paradigm of the diagnosis and treatment of disease, or in the healing, holistic paradigm of naturopathic medicine.

By playing too much in the terrain that is really not our own, we run the risk of becoming obsolete, out-competed by conventional doctors who are highly skilled in allopathic diagnosis and treatment, and who are now adopting many alternative remedies and supplements to complement their practices. The pharmaceutical and neutraceutical industries are paying attention to this interesting new field. What will distinguish us from conventional doctors, if we both practice the "green" way of allopathic medicine? The solution to the dilemma lies in completely embracing the principles of our philosophy, in all elements of our profession and education. We must detach ourselves from all the ways adopted from the allopathic paradigm that do not fit in with the unique, whole person approach naturopathy offers. This will guarantee our role in the medicine of the future.

We face a great challenge. The solution is simple, yet requires much bravery, clarity, and dedication. We must be true to our selves. For the naturopathic profession, this means maintaining our education process in alignment with our philosophy and offering the world our wonderful medicine in its true form, as it was conceived to be. All the credibility and recognition we require will come when we are true to the essence of our medicine and the world sees how gently healing, empowering and cost-effective it really is. We will still graduate properly educated, safe doctors who will do no harm, yet with the roots of our medicine firmly planted in the foundation of Mother Nature. This foundation of our medicine will inspire students to become joyful naturopathic doctors, caring and courageous in the service of humanity.

CHAPTER 1

The 6 Philosophies of Naturopathic Medicine
Introducing the 7th—Physician, Heal Thyself!

Do no harm.
Treat the whole person.
Treat each person as an individual.
Treat the fundamental cause of disease.
Work with the healing power of Nature.
Work as a teacher, facilitator, guide.

CURRENTLY, THERE ARE six different points within the philosophy of our medicine. They are all intimately related and work together to bring about their purpose—to heal people of whatever ailment or condition they may suffer from, whether it is disease that has manifested within the physical body, or mental, emotional dis-ease that has affected the individual. In each healing intervention or act, the naturopathic doctor employs the use of all the philosophies at once. There is no separation between acting as a guide/teacher and working with the healing power of Nature, nor is there a distinction between treating the cause and treating each person as an individual. Equally, when one works with the whole person, he/she is simultaneously practicing all of the other philosophies. The reason for this is because there are not six different points of philosophy—there are simply six points broken down from the *one* essential quality of our medicine—the way of healing.

Since our medicine is a medicine of healing, all other healing professions and disciplines, such as hands-on healing, shamanic healing, and psychotherapy, for example, will recognize the commonalities between our professions and the different ways in which we work to bring healing to the whole person. Thus, our philosophy, though perhaps unique in its expression, is no different from the other forms of healing that have existed for years.

This philosophy is not one person's point of view, nor is it a fleeting fad. Rather, it is the very expression of the healing power of Mother Nature, communicating tenderly how we can return to a state of harmony within ourselves, with all of creation, and how we can reestablish fantastic levels of vitality and well-being. Thus we also recognize that health is not separated from life, so who we are as healers is not separated from who we are as people. In this way, we practice what we preach, and even more importantly, we practice what we are. We also lead by example, demonstrating how our health is intimately related to the way we are living; so much so, that our health is our life. The doctor acts as teacher by personally demonstrating all the benefits of the path of whole person health in harmony with nature.

It is neither wise nor ideal that sick people treat other sick people. Thus, naturopaths and all practitioners who fall within the healing paradigm must heal themselves! This is so fundamentally important that naturopathic medicine will not be able to produce whole NDs until self-healing is made a part of the curriculum. To be a healer, one must go through the process of healing oneself. A naturopath who has gone through his/her healing process has the capacity to provide the necessary space for their copatients[1] to also go through their own healing process.

The healing process does not just involve healing oneself of physical disease, but of all the issues and disharmony one faces in their lives in relationship with themselves, their loved ones and those who grace their lives. All the painful points of our lives, the

---

1. Copatient—A new word for the 'patient' of a naturopath or healer which integrates the fact that there is equality between doctor and patient, thus the prefix 'co'. Copat for short.

issues that trouble us, the burdens that weigh us down can be difficult. The ways in which we are judgmental and non-accepting are also places we must learn to heal ourselves and find a more harmonious way of being, because judgment and healing do not mix. Someone with a sense of peace and who understands the healing process in a non-judgmental manner can provide the right space for a sick, aching person. Otherwise, the situation becomes too uncomfortable, too overwhelming for both the doctor and the copatient. In fact, one who has not embarked upon his/her own healing process is a less effective healer. He/she will have difficulty understanding the subtleties of the healing process, the different expressions of illness in each individual. He/she will be forced to select allopathic solutions with easy formulas. In fact, whether or not a naturopath has learned to heal him/herself might be the most important factor, or even the sole factor, in determining whether he/she will treat the whole copatient naturopathically or whether he/she will treat the symptoms of disease allopathically.

Hypocrites' famous statement, "Physician, Heal Thyself!" should become the 7th Philosophy of Naturopathic medicine because implementing it, carrying it forth within our curriculum, and embodying it amongst our practitioners is crucial for our medicine's well-being and future.

If doctors do not heal themselves, they have less understanding of how to act in conjunction with the points of our philosophy, because each point requires the understanding of the process of healing. To treat each person as an individual, one must be able to understand the unique difficulties, issues, fears and challenges each person faces. This can be very difficult to determine and is a great part of the subtlety of the art of our medicine. The further we are along the path of transformation of our personal growth, the more we can be skilled and sensitive to understand what causes another's disease.

Many people experience great relief following a consultation with a naturopath who is a good listener and is fully present. The ability to be present in an interview and be a good listener is a natural consequence of the process of self-healing. All the stresses and issues that accumulate in an individual weigh them down and pull their awareness inward until they live in their own little world. One might say that self-healing is, therefore, the process by which we remember that we are basically all right and that we need not constantly focus on ourselves. This is why physicians who have healed themselves can be readily present with their copatients.

Healed physicians also run less risk of being "triggered" by their copatients. This is a process that is bound to happen to every practitioner in his/her career; the encounter of people who have such similar issues and patterns of disease and disharmony that they bring up or "trigger" the doctor's own issues. Learning how to deal with one's own issues, one becomes better prepared to understand the internal energetic dance that happens on the healing floor of the practice and how to deal with the resulting emotions.

Treating the fundamental cause of disease comes naturally to the forefront in consultation when we simply provide the space for people to tell us the stories of their lives; their pain and suffering. You, the healer, sitting in a non-judgmental space, are the catalyst that draws out of the person his/her pain and the splinters in his/her mind that cause a cascade of health problems from insomnia, back pain, constipation, migraines, autoimmune disease and cancer.

It is the space that the naturopathic doctor generates from having experienced his/her own healing that provides the proper energy to help another heal. Having experienced the trials of releasing suppressed emotions like sadness and anger, you can then lead another to do the same. Having corrected your eating habits to better serve your body, it is an easy joy to guide others to do the same. Understanding how releasing the limiting belief systems that entrapped you in a certain way of being and made you miserable by dampening your overall well-being, you need only a few additional skills to help guide people in letting go of their limiting belief systems. This is you acting to treat the whole person; spiritually, mentally, emotionally and physically. This is you acting to address the cause of disease (stress, disharmony with oneself and one's environment, negative belief systems, blocked/suppressed emotions) and treating that person as an individual. You have also acted as guide/teacher by helping them find their way by setting an example. By helping your copatients release the stress of their lives, replace the bad foods with good foods, and release toxic thoughts, you act in harmony with the healing power of Nature. Once a dam is released, the waters that nourish the land flow naturally, spontaneously. When you cut yourself, nature heals you when it is unopposed. Understanding this principle, you know the importance of removing not only the obstacles to cure, but the obstacles to life that have caused disease.

Having gone through our own healing process, we get to directly experience and see how mental and emotional stress leads to disease. Being aware of the inner process of healing, we discover how weak we feel when we fear. We observe how greatly our energy changes for the better when we are living according to how we love to be and being ourselves doing what we love to do rather than living the shoulds and musts from our parents, teachers, and leaders. We see how negatively our overall vitality and well-being are affected by our judging, controlling, and worrying.

In 1995, I was diagnosed with the autoimmune disease Myasthenia Gravis (M.G.). I was very sick. I had paralysis of some muscles (triceps, psoas, and abdominal), I had difficulty swallowing, and I was experiencing double vision. I had very little strength and energy and my overall emotional state was very low.

My personal experience with this disease has taught me so much about how and why disease manifests, and about healing. By becoming sick, I learned the ways in which I was not living in harmony with myself and with Nature. Through the years, I have tried many different forms of healing. The form of healing that has always been most effective for me has been self-healing; discovering my issues and fears, learning to let go and be true to myself. I also benefited greatly from homeopathy and a healthy diet. Through my healing process, which is ongoing, I have grown as a person and understand the mind-body connection in health and disease. Having witnessed the healing process upon myself, I trust in it fully.

I have heard people say, "Many patients are just not ready to face their deepest issues." My experience has proven this to be untrue. People are often ready. They are rarely unwilling to face the deep issues that are causing them distress and disease. They might not know it overtly, but inside they are longing to share, to open up and unburden themselves of their issues. Healing is freeing, joyous, and cathartic. It is not something to run in terror from, but to embrace excitedly, willingly. If you fulfill your own healing process, or at least engage that path to some extent, the benefits you have earned from that inner work will be easily conveyed to your copatients, inspiring them to do the same. It is really only a person who has *not* gone through the healing process who claims that people are not ready. They do not trust the healing process. How can you trust anything that you have not personally embarked upon? How can you guide others to do what you have not done yourself?

It is not that people are not ready to embark on their healing process. It is that they are not aware of the wonderful benefits of healing themselves. When people realize what it means to be healthy and well, they become excited by the process and dedicate more of themselves than when they believe that medicine and healing exist simply to patch up health problems when they get out of hand. For this reason, the healed doctor becomes a teacher to awaken people to the magnificence of the healing path.

People come to see you at your practice. In the vast majority of cases, that sets the intention of being ready for healing. It is possible that people are used to the less personal ways of conventional medicine and do not expect to share their whole selves and thus, they come to you just to "fix them." That is your chance to explain how the stresses of their lives and the choices they make cause unhappiness that affects their health. Thus, it is best that they share their issues. It is also a great opportunity to explain the importance of them taking responsibility for their own health. The subject of healing requires a gentle explanation, full of compassion, combined with the clear strength and wisdom that comes from having experienced healing. It doesn't help to have the nervous, apologetic explanation of those who do not trust the path because they are not truly walking it. If you feel sorry and/or apologize for bringing your copatients in the direction of their healing, you are subtly conveying to them that there might be something wrong with that. If you are not sure, how can they be? This sort of attitude must be dismissed so that you can very clearly set the stage for your copatient's health.

It has rarely been the case that my copatients haven't felt comfortable sharing their deepest issues. Many people talk about things they didn't plan to share. It is a natural reaction that occurs between a healer and a copatient. They want to share, they yearn for it, but haven't had the opportunity and or the proper space. When you provide the space to feel comfortable, you also show how important it is to share these deep troubles and buried feelings. (The role of counseling/psychotherapy in naturopathic medicine is escalated because it sets the milieu and serves as the actual engine for connecting deeply with a copatient and for uncovering what is often the cause of disease in these spheres (mental, emotional, and spiritual)).

Dealing with people's health is a challenging enterprise. To have had the gift of knowing, not thinking, not believing, but knowing that the cause of disease originates within the mental and emotional sphere, is a priceless experience that can give you great strength and clarity in dealing with the trials of practicing healing medicine.

I marvel at how people with little experience seeing healers or naturopathic doctors simply accept the way of the healer, as different as it is from the way of the medical doctors, because there is no reason for them not to. Clearly, they expect something different, otherwise they wouldn't seek your help. So give them what they came for, which is being yourself, as different as you may think they perceive that to be. Don't worry about being a flake if you are delving into the mental, emotional, or spiritual. You have studied hard and paid your dues. You have healed yourself, understand how the process works and you know the importance and power of self-healing. You are not a flake. Actually, quite the contrary. You are a brave pioneer in the revolution, not only of naturopathic medicine, but also of the medical world as a whole. Trust that.

Naturopathic medicine should be regarded as different, because it is. It is the new medicine of this age. And because it is different, we should celebrate the difference proudly, gently and bravely. You know the power of healing the whole person. Your lessons were your own healing path, your teacher, your internal wisdom connected with all of Nature. Practicing this form of medicine will also become easier as the groups of people embracing it become larger and more comfortable in public.

Having practitioners who understand the essence of their medicine because they have experienced it firsthand provides an excellent foundation. It also provides a sense of the medicine, an internal knowing and trust that is much better than the cerebral approach of memorizing, studying, and taking written exams. The two ways, when compared, are very different in how effective they are in preparing students to become good naturopathic doctors. We might never be able to prove why healing the whole person and the cause of disease cures. It really doesn't become the number one priority once we have adequately witnessed the healing phenomenon within ourselves.

To experience the healing power of Nature upon oneself, one need not be physically ill. We all have issues, fears, insecurities, illusions about life, judgments, and stresses that keep us out of balance. If a naturopath embarks upon the path to find a better balance in life, with more harmony and vitality, he/she will understand the way of healing. His/her doubts about whole person naturopathy will decrease or cease, even if he/she doesn't have physical disease as a marker. A practitioner who does have his/her own experience of physical or emotional disease gains a phenomenal insight into the healing power of Nature and the way of naturopathic medicine by witnessing his/her own healing process and dealing with the cause of his/her disease.

In order to establish the 7th philosophy in our curriculum and as a profession, we must provide courses designed to help students heal themselves and go through their own processes of transformation. In the Handbook of Accreditation (HOA) for Naturopathic Medicine Programs developed by the Council of Naturopathic Medical Education (CNME), it is written that the core curriculum, "Supports students in becoming empowered primary-care physicians, with a well-developed sense of personal wellness, a knowledge of their unique skills as healers..." p. 43

Thus, the curriculum is responsible for a "well-developed sense of personal wellness" in the students. This, one might say, is similar to, or can be interpreted as, "Physician, Heal Thyself!" Therefore, it is already incorporated into the HOA and must be implemented now with the respective "Physician, Heal Thyself!" courses, which are currently absent from the curriculum.

Naturopathic medicine must be at the cutting edge of the discoveries of consciousness and awareness. Students will come to understand the connection between the choices they make and their health, and between their minds and their bodies. In these classes, students will be encouraged to be themselves, so they can understand how greatly one's health is affected when they do not feel the right to be themselves, and when they make choices outside of who they really are. These classes will also include techniques and methods that are taught in other healing professions that awaken the student's natural abilities of intuition and sensitivity on all levels. Teachers from these other professions could serve as great leaders and guides in the "Physician, Heal Thyself!" courses. Meditation and other exercises that teach the student to be non-judgmental and loving in practice will also be implemented.

There are some healing programs, like *Barbara Brennan's School of Healing,* and other psychotherapy programs that make it an obligatory part of the program that students undergo their own healing process by seeing a psychotherapist once per month, for example, and by giving the students exercises for self-growth and awareness. This too should be included in our curriculum, and is quite simple to implement.

With courses as an integral and required element embedded within our curriculum to carry out the 7th philosophy, (integrated also in courses like psychotherapy and counseling) all students will have the opportunity to understand the essence of our medicine and why it works. Even though the program will continue to challenge, those who chose naturopathic medicine because of its healing philosophy will feel a great joy that they are not being challenged solely to memorize material from a paradigm that is not their own but because they are being challenged to gain the necessary tools to be good healers.

There is another tenet that will serve naturopathic medicine to adopt: "Naturopathic medicine recognizes that responsibility for a person's health is in his/her own hands." Or "Patients are responsible for their own health." This could be adopted as the 8th principle of our medicine, or embraced as a tenet of our philosophy. It is so essential in keeping in harmony with the healing power of Nature and ensuring that naturopathic medicine works with the rest of its philosophy. This additional tenet is discussed in various contexts throughout the book.

CHAPTER 2

The Rational Brain and The Intuitive Mind

If there is any primary rule of science, it is… acceptance of the obligation to acknowledge and describe all of reality, all that exists, everything that is the case… It must accept within its jurisdiction even that which it cannot understand, explain, that for which no theory exists, that which cannot be measured, predicted, controlled, or ordered… It includes all levels or stages of knowledge, including the inchoate,… knowledge of low reliability,… and subjective experience.

—Abraham Maslow

LET'S TAKE A CLOSE LOOK at what science is, how it can be used beneficially in medicine, and how we have often, especially in naturopathic medicine, given our healing abilities and power away by placing too much emphasis on the need to have scientific "proof" and "evidence." When we need to serve science in this way, we are largely misled, as we are confining ourselves in the box of currently established and accepted scientific discovery and principles. This puts us into the pigeonholes of the truth and limits us to practice and view reality in these tight boxes. To place the health of the human being, a vital, fluid, and infinitely complex entity with multiple dimensions, into the current definitions of science and evidence-based medicine does humanity a great disservice.

As accurate as science can be, and as great a tool, it is limited when it comes to being able to sense, detect, and explain the multidimensionality of the human being. We might be technologically very close to detecting the higher levels of the energy field. We already have the capacity to measure and quantify the flow of the acupuncture meridians. Soon there will be devices to detect negative thought forms that begin in the energy field, and to demonstrate how disease then manifests in the physical body. When this occurs, we can use science to technologically serve our understanding of the healing model of whole person medicine. Until and even then, we are best served by the device which has the greatest capacity to detect, understand and work in harmony with the multiple levels of the human being: the intuitive mind of the human being.

The intuitive mind, sometimes called the right brain, is an instrument of many facets and capacities. It is the modem that connects with Nature, downloading material, keeping the human being aware of the present stage. It knows things by a keen sense that is given to us at birth and seems to fade into the furthest reaches of the subconscious when we do not use it or value it. In healing, it is the antenna that feels the deep sadness and woes that people have gone through and detects these disturbances even when they are unwilling or unable to share. It is the intelligence that helps the naturopathic doctor understand the essence behind the creative and fluid modalities we use, like hydrotherapy, homeopathy, acupuncture, and whole person counseling. It is a mind that wraps and bends, retaining a fluid shape capable of grasping the subtleties of natural healing. It is a way of thinking that emerges as people heal and return to a deep connection with themselves and all of nature. The nature doctor who has connection with their intuition and trusts in its power and its mode of action is not concerned at all with what has been proven and what has not. His/her sense of knowing understands principles of healing because it is in direct connection with Nature. To question these principles seems strange and unnecessary, like asking a tree to prove that it needs the sun to survive.

Yet proof, or scientific evidence, is the way we have often sought to carry forward medicine. We wait to walk in the footsteps of scientific discovery, in the law that science has laid down as to what is the truth for our health.

If you really understand what science is, then science at least until now has not been a method for exploring the truth. Science has been a method for exploring our current map of what we think the truth is.

—Deepak Chopra

This approach to healing and medicine is limited because the human being has the capacity to directly intuit and experience the existence of healing principles. Instead of walking in the footsteps of acceptable scientific evidence, we are capable of pioneering the way into the limitless dimensions of reality without needing to look back for permission. Before the word "science" even existed, the healers of the world understood deeply the way of healing and didn't think twice about proving it. Knowing it worked was enough. We have forgotten this way and the deep current of our intuitive nature has been buried beneath another way of thinking.

The need to prove is an act of doubt. When you can connect on the level of awareness with the intuitive mind, which feels out the truth, and you experience that which you can connect with, then there is no need to prove, for you have no doubt. Those people who are able to experience the existence of something, for example, like the feeling or sight of the auric field, or the feeling of the chakras or acupuncture meridians, know beyond doubt that they exist. Even if others are not able to experience it, and doubt the existence, there is no need to prove it. In fact, perhaps ironically, there is no *way* to prove the existence to someone who doesn't feel it or understand within themselves. As in the movie "Contact," the priest asks the doubtful scientist if she loved her father. Her answer is without doubt "Yes." He then says, "Prove it." He makes a brilliant point, since she is skeptical about anything that is not provable scientifically. There is no way to prove she loved her father, but there is also no doubt that she did, so why prove it? More important is the question; "Is it even possible for her to prove it?" I think it is not possible

to prove love exists. For all who experience love and its natural healing powers, does it matter to prove that it exists?

If a group of people enters your naturopathic office and leaves
feeling better, happier and healthier, it doesn't matter what is going
on. It works. You don't have to prove it to the people who feel better.
You also know it works because you did treatment and you chose it
for a reason. Who else is there to prove it to? Thus, our medicine is
empirically based.

Requiring proof and evidence is left-brained in nature—it is
rational. It is all based in past evidence. It works as a kind of backward walking into the steps of the current map that we have accepted
as truth, rather than discovering new worlds by directly experiencing
and experimenting with the realms of the unknown. Most of the civ-
ilized world has become out of balance with too much left-brain
thinking. This way requires proof from the outside to believe, to take
any action, or to use medicine because it is insecure and does not look
to its own inner awareness to find truth. People have taken faith in
science to such a degree that if something has not been established as
truth and accepted collectively by science, people fear it. People can
dismiss something as untrue, not because it *is* untrue, but because it
hasn't been *proven*. Instead of relying on our own intuitive sense of
the truth, which we always have access to, we have given away our
power by asking science to tell us what is acceptable and what is not,
according to what has been proven as truth.

> You see, when science became strong then it eliminated and
> ruled out the true self of humankind, its intuitive self, its self
> of love and heart. It is time for the returning to that, for sci-
> ence placed humankind in holes of pigeons, categorized
> them, labeled them, and put them in a situation such that all
> people began to think of them in that way. Those scientific
> beliefs then led to a pattern of mass thinking.
>
> —*The Only Planet of Choice* p. 287

It is not necessary to *prove* the existence of anything, nor should science ever be employed to validate anything's existence. In order to give ourselves the green light to move forward, all we need to do is *demonstrate* something's validity. What this means is that if it works, it works. This frees us from wasting our time and energy attempting to validate what we do. People have become ingrained in the left-brain, scientific need for proof to such a degree that you can tell them something works, and it has worked on millions of people all over the world for hundreds of years, and they won't believe you unless you can prove it or unless a controlled study has been conducted. This thinking makes no sense. This thinking exists because our society still places immense weight on the "proof first, walk after" approach. It is crippling to live this way because it takes away the human being's ability to know truth by direct connection, by intuitive sense. As long as our medicine is governed by the need for proof approach, we will be carrying out naturopathy in a fearful sort of way, instead of carrying it out bravely and leading others by our example.

The service of humanity that we take an oath to uphold involves many things. As naturopaths, we have a great responsibility to help people remember the intuitive gifts we all have and our capacity to directly know the truth. When our medicine is walking forward into the world demonstrating the truth that is outside of science's pigeonholes, we are fulfilling a very beautiful service for humanity— the healing of false ways of thinking. In that way, we address a large cause of dis-ease in the world that is embedded in medicine and has placed human beings into boxes and treated them as machines.

If we never had perfect evidence to show how homeopathy works, it would still work. If acupuncture remained a total mystery, it would still work. In our scientific arrogance, we dare to question the legitimacy of a medicine that has served people for thousands of years. Why? Because it works in a way that we do not yet understand. Ultimately, we develop the necessary scientific technology to discover why this ancient, incredible medicine works. We just touch

the surface of how it works, and then we make the proclamation—
"There is scientific basis for acupuncture," as if giving it our stamp
of approval legitimizes it.

Imagine if the reign of authorities that lay laws for the "legitimate" practice of medicine began thousands of years ago and even
then required scientific evidence for the credibility of medicine. People would only now be allowed to begin practicing acupuncture.
Homeopathy would barely be accepted (There is evidence for the
scientific validity of homeopathy that is already out there, but it is
undergoing a process of censorship by the authorities of science.
Homeopathy puts many holes into our current map of what we
think the truth is and we can't yet seem to accept that. This is discussed within "*The Memory of Water*" by Michel Schiffe on Jacques
Beneviste's work). Hands-on healing, even today, would still require
many years of scientific advancement before people would be
allowed to practice it. It is absurd when we illustrate these examples
in this way. Yet that is the point. It is absurd to require proof and
evidence of the various aspects of our medicine before we feel completely comfortable embracing and practicing them.

> **Pure logical thinking cannot yield us any knowledge of the
> empirical world; all knowledge of reality starts from experi-
> ence and ends in it.**
>
> —Albert Einstein

Soon we will realize that the need to know and prove comes from
the need to be in control. That need comes from the fear of being out
of control, thus we have forced ourselves and our beliefs upon Nature
in an attempt to make ourselves feel in control. Soon we will come to
accept that one cannot order the truth into a scientific formula that is
fixed in any permanent way, especially for our health. Everyone is different and the reason why people get sick is unique to each individual.
That being true, the way to help those individuals return to health is

also unique to them and will not ever be perfectly reproducible, no matter how technologically advanced we become.

It is therefore impossible to attempt to validate naturopathic medicine, homeopathy, acupuncture, or any other subtle medicine that works with the healing power of Nature by performing, for instance, double-blind studies. These studies prove nothing in whole person naturopathic medicine because each person is unique and disease has manifested for different reasons according to each case. Remember the expression, "One person's potion, another person's poison?" In the healing paradigm, you cannot reproduce a scientifically-sound method that is going to help all people. Yet this is one reason why healing medicines are frowned upon by the left-brain of science—because they work in ways that cannot be carved in stone, nor reproduced for others to emulate. And therefore our responsibility to the world is to explain how this approach to medicine does not really cure people of their ailments in a way that serves to bring balance and health to all levels of their being. Our role is not to attempt to validate our medicine through scientific methods like double-blind study, but rather to show people that such methods of proof and evidence treat every person the same way—symptomatically, mechanistically, and according to the disease, and yet, we are truly all different. Equally, our role becomes to nurture the new way of whole person healing, where all people are shown their responsibility for their own health and taught not to be afraid to trust their intuitive abilities.

The doubt that we may have about how the world will respond to our new and unproven medicine makes us look for proof to feel secure that we too can reproduce a method or a technique. Insecurity makes people look to prove themselves, just as teens who wish to be accepted into the in-crowd make great attempts to prove themselves in order to be accepted. This is a mistake as it only serves to alienate people even more from who they are. And even if the efforts to prove oneself work to win access to the in-crowd, that act of gaining acceptance comes with a very high price—the price of selling out who the person really is. Their efforts to gain acceptance are not in being who they are but in emulating the way of the in-crowd. The mistake is seen especially when realizing that in order to remain a part of the in-crowd, they must continue acting the way that enabled them to gain access in the first place.

Naturopaths do not want to be accepted into the in-crowd of established scientific medicine because that would require selling out the essence of our medicine, which will bind us to that way as long as we continue to seek its acceptance. This quick way of seeking credibility is the lesser choice for the profession in the long run. And by seeking acceptance in a model of medicine that is not in harmony with the healing power of Nature, we are making a statement to the world that we believe this is the correct way because we are seeking entrance into it. That too is an error.

All we can do is develop our naturopath skills in the various modalities we work with, continue to grow in treating the whole person, and improve ourselves at helping people get to the causes of their dis-ease. We must get all of these skills down to a "science." That is what our science is, and it is a way that will attract all the credibility we need, because it works. The world is ready for this medicine in its pure form. And we will be like the teen who didn't seek quick acceptance but rather slowly blossomed into his/her own person and found the reward in living that way; by being true to one's self.

Naturopaths are skilled in the science of their unique expression of healing, just as they work with each person as an individual. But is it an exact science? No. It is an individual's science, a skill used creatively and specially in every case, and that cannot be taught in an absolutely reproducible manner. They might use homeopathy, counseling, and nutrition to help their copatients heal. They might use tuning forks or drums, dance therapy, music therapy or light therapy. Whatever a healer aligns with, whatever he/she feels inspired to practice, that is his/her way, skill, and science. And if it works and you don't know why, give thanks that it works and turn off that pesky voice that needs an answer for everything.

Taking something apart in order to understand it is like splitting atoms. One can keep splitting forever. This is like throwing rocks into the Grand Canyon. This is the dilemma science faces today, especially the biomedical scientific approach to our health. Looking deeper and deeper at the body as a series of genetic transcriptions, the expression of proteins, and all the interactions between the cells' communication, one can continue to pull apart ad infinitum, looking for the way it all comes together. This is a never-ending process leading to a dead end. The reality is so much simpler.

The right brain of healing and the intuitive mind are aligned with the simple truth. It is so simple that it naturally sheds formulas and definitions until it boils itself down into a powerful, undefined essence. Yes, there is truth. It heals us and brings us clarity and a sense of purpose. It makes us live. Yet we cannot define it or explain exactly what it is. We know that it is there, but we might never be able prove it, which might be a blessing in disguise. We cannot say for sure what the healing power of Nature is, nor what the innate intelligence of life is, Gaia. That helps it remain a mystery so that we cannot get our hands all over it and try to fix it to a definition. That way it remains pure. All we will ever be able to do is experience this essence, both by being ourselves and through the practice of our healing medicine. In serving Mother Nature by the subtle art of nature cure, She serves us in a mysterious way whose ultimate evidence is better health in the people whom She touches.

The way of the Tao is not the eternal way.
It cannot be defined or explained.
It can only be experienced.

—Anonymous

The healing way of our philosophy, much like the way of Taoism, must never be concrete and defined. Yes, there is an essence to it; a path, so to speak. It is the philosophy of our medicine. But once on the path, you can dance your medicine, drum it, whistle to heal people, clap your hands, use homeopathy, herbs, acupuncture, bells and whistles, or whatever, as long as you're treating the whole person, as individuals, in the root of their disease, and in harmony with Mother Nature.

It just so happens that under the canopy of naturopathic medicine, there are a few modalities and methods of treatment that we do learn, such as homeopathy, acupuncture, Bowen, and cranio-sacral therapy that have not yet been entirely proven scientifically. This too might be a blessing in disguise because these beautiful and very effective modalities might never catch the disease that so many disciplines do—the disease of making solid definitions and then becoming stuck to serve the definitions rather than serving the essence behind the discipline.

The great homeopaths of today are paving the way into new territory, expanding the medicine by incorporating fresh ideas and implementing them effectively in practice. This is progress. The new and improved homeopathy is based upon the essence of the old, but is not restricted to old definitions that would otherwise limit it. People, who have interpreted the medicine to be a certain way and require it to be that way and not any other way, have fallen in the trap of the left-brain, which cannot see beyond the definitions it has accepted as true. This is backward stagnation and does not keep up with the ever-changing rhythms of the world.

"The reasonable person adapts themselves to the world.
The unreasonable person persists in trying to adapt the world to themselves.
Therefore all progress depends on the unreasonable person."
—George Bernard Shaw

Naturopathic medicine must pave the way, readily growing and accommodating the demands of society's sick. To do so, we must also help the world change by encouraging the model of healing that is our own, and not by trying to adapt to the world as it is now. Much of this healing must take place in our colleges, which have been heeding an obligation to adapt to the way of established medicine. This is a reflection of the method of thinking that is "proof-first, change after" that obviously affects not only science and medicine, but has found its way into our corridors.

Another good reason to remain Nature doctors and to seek the longer road of acceptance in being true to the self is to remember that in the attempt to control the nature of reality, people have become controlling toward one another. As naturopaths, it is important for us to be aware that in the world of medicine, people do attempt to control the expression of other people's medicine. The authorities on medicine have tried to dictate what goes and what does not, and the method with which they establish what is acceptable is through scientific evidence that makes a machine out of the body, which is disconnected from the mind, and has created many belief systems about who we are. This is controlling because it allows neither the existence of other points of view, nor different expressions of the healing power of Nature. Rather, it takes away our ability to tap into the infinite potential of the healing power of Nature, sometimes by censorship and the imposition of unfair laws, such as the banning of healing substances, or sometimes worse.

Guylaine Lanctôt, a medical doctor from Quebec, for fear of her life, had to go into hiding to write her book, "The Medical Mafia," which reveals shocking truths about the system we have called "Health Care." According to Lanctôt, there is little care in the system for our health, for it is run by an industry that profits from our disease. Lanctôt risked her career and her life to write this book and paint us the picture of her understanding of the multidimensionality of the human being and how each level, not just the physical, must be addressed.

Lanctôt also described her awareness of truths that she did not learn in school. She discussed the human being's ability to use intuition and spoke of her own ability, which awakened once she accepted that which is beyond the rational.

> There is no need to go outside for better seeing, nor to peer from a window. Rather abide at the centre of your being, for the more you leave, the less you learn.
>
> —Lao Tse Tao Te Ching

What this quotation means is that we have an inherent ability, without going outside ourselves or into books, to heal, especially if we have the wish to heal others and we embark on own our healing path. But our society is structured not to encourage this way of being, nor to support those people who have the gift of the healer. What is required of people who want to be naturopathic healers today is that they go through a rigorous and rigid form of education that is entirely left-brained and rational. This sets up an illusion of credibility and maintains the control of the left brain in medicine.

Because our society is still so rational, and because there still does exist the threat of censorship and legal control over certain medicines, it therefore makes sense that we have some fear of carrying out our healing medicine in the true and pure form. The rational, left-brain is a Yang/male energy. The Yin/female aspect is aligned with the right brain, the way of intuition, and the undefined way. It is no wonder that over 70% of practitioners of healing medicines, including hands on healing, naturopathy, homeopathy, and many others, are women, because these medicines have their essence in, and are most effective with, their foundation in the intuitive.

Through the centuries, the female aspect of humanity has been attacked and dominated by the patriarchy. This has manifested in many ways, for example, by the churches' burning of millions of so-called "witches" at the stake for practicing what simply could have been herbal medicine or other forms of healing that were considered outside the accepted norm of the Church. The male aspect has dominated religion through the rational approach to God and the judgment and association of Eve/Lilith as being evil and consorting with the Devil. The domination of the female aspect of healing still occurs today on a large scale in most societies. Even in our naturopathic schools, the rational approach is dominant, and the intuitive approach and the undefined way of our philosophy is still given little attention.

We are afraid to be called witches and voodoo magic users, either because of the memories we have of the healers and witches being burned at the stake, or because of the still-present threat that the medical mafia and the left brain impose on the healing world. But there is absolutely no way that this can continue if the naturopathic profession, *in strength of numbers and as the strength of a profession*, overcomes this fear of being out in the world as a healing-based medicine. This book calls us to play a large role in bringing the intuitive mind, the way of the female healing energy, back into the world, to be accepted and supported by the government and the people.

The suppression of the Yin/female way of healing has occurred whether it has been in a man or a woman. Men and women are comprised both of the male and female energies—Yin and Yang. The Church also burned men at the stake if they were considered "wise men" or "warlocks," or if they were found to associate with any mystical practice or connection with nature that was not understood or practiced by the Church. Whoever it may be who practices the female way of medicine, is considered a threat to the person who is governed by their left-brain.

The basis for our medicine should be in the right brain, with the undefined, intuitive way serving as the foundation. This does not, however, mean to indicate that one should throw their left brain into the garbage, or that only women have the necessary skills to be healers. To have the balance of the left and right brains is incredibly powerful and essential in the practice of healing and medicine. How this is done might not be as one would expect. The left brain must ultimately serve the right brain, just as science can serve us in healing, and just as in Chinese medicine the Yang organs carry forward the essence created in the Yin organs. This creates harmony.

The right brain is the intuitive connection between healer and copatient and the receiver of the vital information of the case. The left brain brings forth understanding of the information gleaned from the copatient in order to select a course of treatment. The right brain establishes the connection with a copatient and grants intuitive awareness of what is blocked, what is out of balance, what is the cause, and what is unique to this individual. This becomes the foundation for the action of the left brain to have a sense of what to do with all that info, for example, what modalities to apply, what remedy, acupuncture needle, diet change, etc., that will bring forth healing. However, even the understanding that the left brain has in a case of what to do comes from the right brain's intuitive awareness. The right brain is the quarterback who hands off the ball to the left brain, who carries it forward. The right brain is an open connection with the communication of Nature that reveals to you each case's uniqueness, conveying to you in the interview what are the important points to focus on. It is the guidance from Nature's healing power of the right brain that reaches down into your left brain and pulls the string, lighting the closet containing the learned information that will help your case. It is a sense conveyed to you, not one that you must figure out. Physicians/healers often have a spontaneous intuitive sense of what to do in a case, and what is most important. If this is questioned by the rational mind, "Are you sure? Where is the evidence for that choice?" it interferes with the spontaneous process of direct knowing. (These references to left and right brain are only intended metaphorically for the rational (left) and intuitive (right) methods of thought. The left brain is not always rationally dominant, especially in left-handed people).

Naturally, it is very helpful to develop knowledge in the modalities one is using. Knowing all that one can know about homeopathy and acupuncture, for instance, is very useful in practice. This is the left brain's territory. Practitioners must always be flexible with the information they learned so that they don't start projecting their knowledge onto their copatients, or they will not be respecting, "Treat each person as an individual." In homeopathy, this becomes evident when the practitioner knows a limited number of remedies and attempts to place the copatient into one of those remedies. Someone exhibits loquacity, jealousy, and suspiciousness and the practitioner thinks of Lachesis, since this is the remedy they know. This is almost like treating the disease. This is a way of practicing that is based in the foundation of the left brain. This is not working in harmony with the healing power of Nature, which involves being all ears and having completely open eyes to listen and observe all that the copatient shares with you. By being in this blank, receptive state, you might discover that what this person is really trying to tell you, without even expressing it overtly, is that he/she has never recovered from a horrible, fearful shock experienced years earlier. You sense that underneath the copatient's outward expression. They are telling you they need the remedy aconitum. Of course, in order to give aconitum, you have to know about it. Yet when a course of treatment is shown by the subconscious of the copatient and conveyed to you upon the subtle channels of Nature, that is the most powerful way of practicing.

In the long run, a person who develops the skills to be completely receptive to allow the healing power of Nature to work through them (developed largely through the process of self-healing) is more equipped to heal the whole person. Who really knows what a person needs? Only that person and Nature do. He/she might need to listen to a bird's song, or to enjoy the pleasures of sex. The practitioner can know too, but only by *receiving* the information, on all levels, provided by the copatient. The physician who has developed his/her knowledge is very useful—the more knowledge, the better. Yet if he/she applies too much knowledge, rather than observation, the relationship with Nature is not in harmony. The doctor is still too much in control.

That is one of the scary aspects of whole person healing and Nature cure. Each case is unique. There are no references points where one can flip to a page and be told what to do. You're on your own, so to speak—just you, the copatient, and Nature. That is why it is so essential to develop the intuitive mind. It is the intelligence of Nature, fluid and creative, taking on whatever form necessary.

Moving the foundation of healing medicine back onto Mother Earth, into the intuitive and simple realm where the healing power of Nature naturally occurs, brings back to the practitioner the feeling and knowledge of his/her innate ability to heal. This knowing comes even without having learned any particular skills. This power of healing can emerge from a person in a way that is very surprising. If one's entire foundation is stacked upon the need for evidence and the need to learn from the outside, one will lack trust in his/her own abilities to intuit the truth and connect to one's inner power of healing. There is a lot of insecurity in the "needing to rely on knowledge" way because one has not developed intuitive knowing. If one is amongst many people who live believing that one's worth, in healing, for instance, is valued by how much one *knows*, as in how much text book knowledge one has, then a person can look at themselves and say, "I do not know these things, I must not be good enough." This way of thinking has its foundation in the rational and evidence-based approach to medicine. It forgets the simple truth that healing abilities are inherent and can often emerge with no external learning. If children, who exhibited gifts of intuitive insight and a natural wish to help others, were encouraged to trust their instincts, they would be very powerful healers, without learning any additional skills.

As naturopaths who allow the intuitive way of medicine back into our medicine, in practicing what we know works and what we know to be true, even if there isn't scientific evidence for it, we will then get all the recognition we need. If we are true to ourselves, the public will seek our help. Soon, there will be too many miracles of cure happening at the hands of the healing paradigm for even the most doubtful person not to be affected and roused into wakefulness. Have faith that what you do is good and let go of the need to prove yourself. You are a healer. Let science serve you, if you wish. You don't have to serve science. The general public and the government will see this as well when we, the healers and those who live within that narrow margin where the intuitive and undefined are a part of everyday life, stop trying to prove ourselves, have faith and practice our medicine freely in the world.

Then we can begin to really use the science of nature to move forward with the amazing work of people like Royal Rife (Rife Beam Ray Devices; known to cure cancer in the 1940s and 1950s), Jacques Beneviste, Wilhelm Reich, and many others. Reich's orgone technology is a world of limitless possibilities and immense potential. We could delve into this world and further study and expand the principles of the universal life energy (orgone/ki/qi/prana), how to accumulate it, harness it, and use it for healing, fuel for transportation, and other phenomenal applications. As naturopaths dedicated to the service of humanity, and as Lust's stated, our "worldwide purpose," we are not meant to simply heal copatients one on one. We are meant to heal the planet, its faulty thinking, polluted transportation system, and failing economy. There are people today harnessing the power of the orgone energy, building energy cells that power cars. Called the "Joe Cell," after the Australian man who created it, these fuel cells are running cars on simply the "free energy" of the universe. There are no by-products, no waste, no pollution. Imagine the changes that implementing such a technology alone could have on the planet. Think of the oil industry, its pollution, its war on the world for domination. Think of what an amazingly better world we could live in if we helped forward such technology. This work most definitely falls into the world of science, yet can move forward at alarming rates of discovery and expansion of knowledge without being tied to the trap of EBM and the elimination of the empirical. From this angle, one can observe that EBM and the science that falls into that fishbowl, actually slows the discovery of technology in the direction that can help the planet.

I see a vision of our medicine doing research into these fields of orgone energy, and on the human energy field, chakras, and acupuncture meridians, on light and sound healing, brain-balancing technology, and much more. And then using our knowledge of the body, acupuncture meridians, and chakras, to further the efficiency of the modalities and technologies we use to heal our copatients. If naturopathic medicine reunites with its roots, trusting in the healing power of Nature without need for immediate recognition from established science and medicine, we will have departments in our colleges to do research into these amazing worlds, waiting to be discovered and employed. Then, working with the undeniably incredible technologies of orgone energy, Joe cell, Rife Beam Ray Devices, etc., and marrying those to our medicine's knowledge, people will no be longer worry about having proof. It will be right before their eyes.

CHAPTER 3

Naturopathy's Gift of the Mind-Body Connection

Pythagoras said that the most divine art was that of healing.
And if the healing art is most divine, it must occupy itself
with the soul as well as with the body; for no creature can be
sound so long as the higher part in it is sickly.

—Apollonius of Tynana

PEOPLE HAVE CALLED naturopathic doctors, "Jacks of all trades,
masters of none." Other professions specializing in their own treatment modality, such as chiropractors, herbalists, or homeopaths,
have criticized naturopathy because of this eclecticism. Yet having
access to the knowledge of so many different medicines, philosophies, and scientific knowledge, naturopathic medicine has a special
ability to unify these different theories and philosophies with science, to demonstrate the connection of the mind and body in healing. By providing the bridges that show how they all relate and
interconnect, we have the potential to explain and demonstrate how
disharmonies in the mind and emotions result in disease in the body.

Keeping with the essence of the previous chapter, this unification
and explication of whole person medicine might not yet be accepted
into current scientific theory. This doesn't indicate that we are incapable of understanding based on our current knowledge of healing and
science. It just means that it hasn't yet been accepted. In the future,
there might be technology to demonstrate all of the philosophy in this
chapter. Before then, we can help make it acceptable by trusting in it
ourselves and then by sharing it with the public with clear examples
and good analogies. The naturopath and healer, having trust in the

treatment modalities that the profession offers, doesn't require absolute proof of the common vein that runs through many of our healing modalities and philosophies. It is at our fingertips to personally experience and understand by intuitive and empirical confirmation. We have a model to remind us that there is a connection between the mind and the body. We have a model that can help uncover many of the mysteries of holistic medicine. And then we can further carry out our role in society as "Doctor as Teacher" by providing this model to our copatients to help them understand their own healing processes.

Let us take a look at the gift that naturopathic medicine has in providing the whole picture in whole person medicine. We will dip into the wells of knowledge of acupuncture and Traditional Chinese medicine, hands on healing, homeopathy, chiropractic, counseling and psychotherapy, physiology and anatomy, and other medicines and scientific knowledge.

The Three Treasures in Chinese Medicine states that the Mind (Shen) governs the Energy (Qi) which governs the Blood (Jing). Blood is the Three Treasure's equivalent to the body. By "governs," it means that the mind can control the flow of the Qi, through the acupuncture meridians, which controls the flow of the blood in the body. When the Qi stops flowing, the blood stops flowing. Once that has occurred, disease begins to manifest in the physical body.

There are two questions to address now—

HOW does the mind control the Qi?
WHY does the mind control the Qi?

First, let's look at HOW. For this, we can examine the relationship between the mind and the chakras, and how the chakras have their influence on the acupuncture meridians and Qi.

There are seven chakras situated on the body. The term "chakra" is a Sanskrit word meaning "wheel." Some people have the ability to see the chakras, the acupuncture meridians, and even the levels of the energy field surrounding the body, called the aura. Barbara Brennan is a gifted healer who has an amazing ability to see the different levels of the auric field and the chakras. In her books, *Hands of Light* and *Light Emerging*, she describes in remarkable detail the chakras and the different levels of the human energy field. She describes the chakras as funnels of energy that draw in and absorb the universal life energy that we have called Qi (Chinese), Ki (Japanese), Prana (Sanskrit), and Orgone (a term by Wilhelm Reich). I have seen the chakras appear as funnels as well. The Qi/life energy that the chakras provide us from the Universe nourishes our systems with the energy we need to live and be healthy. The Qi that is drawn in through the chakras then passes into the acupuncture meridians, just as lakes and oceans provide the source of water for rivers and streams. These wheels/chakras exist at a high vibrational frequency, so we are generally unable to detect them with the naked eye unless we have developed our high sensory perception or we are able to see high frequencies with the third eye—the chakra situated on the forehead between our eyes. Today, very sensitive low-light cameras and Kirlian photography are able to capture on film the chakras and some of the levels of the auric field.

The seven chakras can be categorized by pairs of front and rear chakras, which have a Yin and Yang relationship with each other. The front chakras are Yin in nature; female, because they are the feeling chakras and they are afferent, meaning that they receive the energy from the Universe and we can only allow their flow to occur, we cannot control it. The rear chakras are Yang in nature; male, because they are the will chakras and are efferent in nature. Through the rear chakras we can control the flow of our energy with our will.

In Chinese medicine, it is said that the Yin organs create the precious and vital fluids and essences of our bodies and the Yang organs store the precious energies or carry them out to fulfill their functions in the body. The same is true of the chakras. The Yin chakras provide all the nourishment of our body by receiving the universal life energy. The Yang chakras function to bring forth that energy we receive through the Yin chakras to nourish the body. The balance of Yin and Yang in this relationship is vital for the health of the human being. The energy that the chakras provide through the acupuncture meridians nourishes the various nerve plexuses, organs and tissues of the body in the region of that chakra. The blood follows the flow of Qi. When the Qi flows, the blood is invigorated and brings health to the region of the body it supplies. This happens as naturally as the flow of a stream down a mountain. It requires very little input from our own will. In fact, as we will see, it is when we try too hard to control, that our energetic systems become dis-eased.

> The powerful flow of life-force that comes with the involun-tary divine creative principle cannot be commanded by the ego. Another way to say this is that the goodness within you flows of its own accord; it reaches out in wisdom, love, and caring of its own accord. It does not flow on the command of the ego. The only thing the ego can do is stop it from flowing or get out of its way.
> — Barbara Ann Brennan, Light Emerging, p. 265

There are four levels of reality in the human being. In naturo-pathic medicine, we describe these as the spiritual, mental, emo-tional, and physical realms. The upper three levels are solely energetic in nature. Even the physical body is made up of energy that we perceive as something solid and dense because of its slow vibrational frequency. It is made up of molecular structures and cells that are the building blocks that give the human being, and all phys-ical matter, form. The subatomic particles that make up these build-ing blocks of matter are also energetic in nature. It is on the physical realm that the Blood, from the Three Treasures, flows.

As the vibrational frequencies of the energy and matter that make up the human being increase, the result is more difficult to perceive with our eyes, as we discussed with the chakras.

The chakras and the meridians where the Qi flows make up the next realm, higher in vibrational frequency than the physical realm. This emotional realm does not simply contain our emotions, but is also the level of reality in the human being that contains the chakras and the acupuncture meridians. Our emotions are also called our feelings because the emotional realm contains the feeling chakras, which give rise to what we perceive as our feelings. In the Three Treasures, this is the level of Qi. Since the Qi is on a higher level than the physical body (Blood), it governs and influences the body.

The next level, higher in energetic frequency, is the mind; the mental realm. It is difficult to see this level, even with high sensory perception. It is also called "the level of intention" by Barbara Brennan. Our mind is responsible for the intentions that we think, speak, and carry out in action. The mind's intention is the same as our will. We carry out this will in the emotional realm through the rear chakras and in the physical realm through our efferent nervous system, which controls our muscles.

Here is HOW the mind controls the flow of Qi. Since the rear chakras are the will centers, they are governed by the intention of the mind. What we intend, therefore, influences the flow of the chakras. Through the will chakras, we have the ability to control the flow of the feeling chakras. The will chakras can act as a brake to stop or slow the flow in the receptive, nourishing feeling chakras. We do this all the time with our emotions, or our feelings, by blocking the feelings that we do not like to experience. This prevents the proper energizing in those areas of the body nourished by the chakras.

Here we enter the world of counseling and psychotherapy to explain WHY the mind controls the Qi, which will provide us a great link in the picture of whole person medicine.

Quite simply, this has everything to do with our beliefs about reality. Our beliefs about reality are called "belief systems." Belief systems are concepts and ideas that we have about reality that we hold on to, sometimes cling on to, because we believe we must. In homeopathy, we call these belief systems "delusions." They are delusions because we believe something about reality that is not necessarily true or accurate, even though to us it has the appearance of truth.

It is not that we *have* beliefs that it makes us sick. If people believe that love is a powerful healing energy, this does not limit them or cause disharmony in their systems. It is when they NEED to believe certain things and have attachments to their ideas that they become sick. Rigidly holding on to fixed belief systems creates disease. Rigidity is the antithesis of life.

We hold on to these beliefs/delusions because we feel they fulfill some ultimate function in our lives, like helping us deal with the pain of life, the loss of love, to justify a harsh reality or to protect us from our fears. A child who learns that he/she needs to become obsequious to gain approval and affection (experienced as love) from his/her parents, will grow up believing that being obsequious earns love. In fact, it will be difficult for the child not to be obsequious in relationships, because the two go hand in hand. People who have been put down in their lives because they didn't conform with the norm, might hold on to the belief that it is not safe to be themselves to avoid the pain of rejection.

Whatever their belief system, human beings feel they must maintain what they have adopted as truth or else they feel their reality is being threatened. It gives us a sense of security to see that what we believe to be true is confirmed in reality. When someone's belief system is challenged, he/she reacts as if something bad has happened. His/her reality is being challenged or threatened. If you grow up believing that people shouldn't show their bellies in public, you will be triggered to feel that something bad is happening when you witness someone's belly being exposed publicly. If you believe that you are royalty and should be treated that way, your reality will feel threatened and you will experience the event as bad when someone treats you in a way that you perceive as unworthy.

The unhealthy response to our belief systems being threatened is to attempt to control our reality. This happens in various ways and to various degrees. Some people would respond to the bare belly by scoffing and walking away, or by avoiding looking at the belly altogether. Others might try to control the situation by insisting that the person cover the belly. For the person who believes they are royalty, all situations and people that do not fulfill their belief about reality will be met with a response that will attempt to eliminate the situation or person from their reality. All negative, "bad!" responses to no-bare belly, I am royalty, or any other belief systems, are acts of control.

Putting a "bad" label on something is a judgment. When you judge something as bad, you are acting as judge over reality, and you become controlling because you are not allowing that thing that you judge as bad to exist. Everything in the Universe that is judged reacts by trying to prove it is worthy of existence. So even for those things which we all agree are not what we want to live with, like pain and dis-ease, by judging them as bad, we fight against them and thus give them a place in our bodies. The battle we take against something that we view as bad actually encourages it to exist because of all the focus on it. The response of a wise person, which is healing in nature, is to accept all things in reality and then create reality according to how one would love to have it. The response of acceptance is very powerful to help transform our health and the world around us. By not focusing too harshly or judgmentally on that which we do not want to have in our world, these things dissipate and people have a choice to adopt a new way of being.

By judging something as bad, and acting to eliminate it from our reality, we elicit a controlling reaction inside of us. In the emotional realm, because we say "No" or "Bad" to the situation, we will put out our mind's intention to use the will chakras to stop the flow of the feeling chakras. This is the process by which a negative emotion or feeling is generated. The feeling chakras feel good to us when they are allowed to be. When we resist and try to control our reality, the will centers get in the way of this natural flow process and impede it. And so when we judge a situation as bad and decide we must be in control, the extra will we use to be in control interferes with the natural flow of the feeling chakra and creates a negative feeling. In addition to the negative feeling that is generated, there is a lack of the positive feeling that is naturally provided by the feeling chakra. So reality will begin to feel and appear negative, which is a kind of confirmation of the original judgment that led to the resistance of the feeling chakra. This is the energetic explanation of projection.

The eye sees what it brings to seeing.

—Percy Shelley

With this control, there will also be a lack of nourishment of the body from that feeling chakra. The balance of the acupuncture meridians will be affected, the flow of Qi disturbed, which will ultimately result in the decrease of flow of the blood to the regions of the body supplied by that chakra. This results in physical disease.

When the mind lives in the confinements of certain belief systems, it usually affects the specific chakras related to the issues of those belief systems. Naturally, the related parts of the body are also affected. For example, a person who has low self-esteem and fears failure forms beliefs like, "I am no good. I can't get anything right" or, "I am stupid" and can develop digestive disorders because the solar plexus chakra (third chakra) is affected. The third chakra, located on the solar plexus, is related to our feeling of self-esteem and our confidence to be ourselves. This chakra nourishes the liver, spleen, pancreas and stomach, as well as the nerve plexus, the muscles, tissues and bones of the surrounding areas. In situations where someone who believes, "I can't get anything right," is required to perform, he/she will be very hard on him/herself. Instead of the natural, carefree and effective way of people who feel good about themselves, the way of the insecure person becomes strangulated or stressed in their attempts to perform effectively. They drive through their lives with one foot on the gas, trying to accomplish their work, and one foot on the brake (the will chakras saying "No, I can't"), believing they are incapable of success. Everything will be a big deal for them, and there will be lots of worry. Since the solar plexus chakra nourishes the stomach, it is no wonder that many people who lack self-esteem develop stomach problems ranging from heartburn and ulcers to stomach cancer.

We also tend to judge emotions that we attempt to control with our will. The suppression of the flow of emotions is a big problem for our health and is at the root of many chronic diseases. When someone suffers the loss of a loved one, at times the grief seems overwhelming. If he/she does not mourn properly, he/she will try to stop his/her feelings. The whole grieving experience is viewed as bad and the person uses his/her intention from the mind to force the will chakra to stop the feeling. Sadness is experienced in the lungs. The lungs are nourished by the heart chakra since they are in the region that is supplied life energy by the heart chakra. Love connections are also experienced in the heart chakra. The painful detachment of connections from the loss of a loved one, felt in the front, feeling heart chakra and the lungs, will be resisted by a mind that judges the feeling of grief as bad. When the person says either subconsciously or consciously "No!" to the feeling of grief, the rear, will heart chakra is used to stop the feelings.

What can result from this suppression of the front feeling chakra from grief is any number of health problems. In homeopathy, we would call this, "ailments from grief" or "ailments from disappointed love." The person can develop anxiety and/or depression because the great feeling of strength and calm that comes from the properly-functioning heart chakra has been compromised. The person can have postural problems because the grief bends them over, resulting in kiphosis. The muscles become weakened in the thoracic region supplied by the heart chakra, so the musculature can no longer support the skeletal structure, and the person bows over with time. There can be serious problems of the immune system, since the lungs are the source of the Wei Qi, which is the defensive energy that protects the body from external pathogens. The thymus gland, where the T lymphocytes go through their maturation process, also gets its nourishment from the heart chakra. So when the heart chakra energy is weak, the immune system is weakened. Naturally, the heart is affected by a blocked heart chakra. Any number of heart conditions can result. On a more general level, if the heart isn't strong, its action on the blood is lessened and the pumping of the blood throughout the body is lessened. This greatly affects the person's entire system. Blood pressure and circulation problems, muscular weakness, aching and overall fatigue can result. The decreased flow of blood to the brain can cause memory problems, poor concentration and focus, and decrease in alertness. The overall experience of life is affected from an under-functioning heart. This all stems from the resistance of the mind.

A grief-stricken person can present with any or all of the above complaints. In practice, it is not uncommon for someone to present with chronic fatigue and fibromyalgia, depression, anxiety, insomnia, indigestion, constipation, back pain, headaches and memory problems. These can all be chronic manifestations of the person not dealing properly with the loss of a loved one. Imagine the green allopathic approach in such a case and all of the problems simply originate from the mental emotional sphere. Tolle Causum. Treat the cause and you will solve most health problems.

Our society has a lot of judgments surrounding sex. The chakra that is associated with our sexuality is the second chakra, located just below the navel. It nourishes the surrounding area including the bladder, the pelvis and the sexual organs. Someone who has developed a belief system that sex is bad will judge their sexual feelings and learn to suppress them on command of their will. What can result are ailments from suppressing the sexual desire, to use the homeopathic rubric. These ailments could eventually lead to impotence, premature ejaculation, prostatitis or prostate cancer in men, menstrual disorders, dysparenuia, ovarian cysts or uterine fibroids, and any sort of cancer seen in the pelvis, in woman. Bladder problems could also manifest in a person who attempts to suppress sexual feelings. The second chakra is also related to how we feel about ourselves. The negative feelings in relation toward ourselves can generate a sense of self-loathing and ugliness which can lead to low self-esteem, self-deprecation and destruction, depression, auto-immune disease, possible eating disorders like anorexia and bulimia, and many other conditions that result from a person's lack of self-love.

The second chakra can also begin to malfunction when a person develops belief systems about themselves being bad, or ugly, or unclean from the people in their environment. If someone is told repeatedly, "You are ugly" or, "You're no good. What's the matter with you?" one of the ways he/she might respond is by controlling the flow of the second chakra. This will help create emotions in the way they believe themselves to be—bad, ugly, no good. Through the manifestation of disease, the body will continue the process the mind has begun, having adopted negative or limiting belief systems about itself.

It would greatly benefit the people we contact, through treatment and educational lectures and seminars, to make it known that suppressing emotions leads to disease. Allowing one's emotions to flow keeps one in a state of calm, restores the proper balance of one's energetic system, and empowers the nourishing action of the feeling chakras. When people know this and apply it to themselves, they become better equipped to deal with their own health. They have restored the relationship between their mind, body and health, are less dependent on their doctors to fix them, and we have thus fulfilled part of our role as teachers of Nature's healing ways.

In the physical realm, our autonomic nervous system is the physical parallel of our chakra system on the emotional level.

The parasympathetic nervous system is necessary for proper digestion of food, for elimination, and for the healing of the body. It is active during times when there is no stress and worry. It is Yin in nature and is therefore parallel to the front, feeling chakras.

The sympathetic nervous system is necessary to awaken the body into an active state, during times of rigorous physical activity, when the heart pumps lots of blood and the lungs are breathing in larger volumes of oxygen. When the sympathetic nervous system is active, the body is generally in an "on-guard" state and the muscles are ready for action. It is the response to stressful situations. That is why it is called the "Fight or Flight" nervous system of the body. The sympathetic nervous system suppresses the immune system. When you are running for your life, your body doesn't focus on your immune system's defense, or healing. You need to be in control. The sympathetic nervous system is Yang in nature.

When a belief system is triggered, the result is identical to a stress response. This is the case no matter what the belief system and regardless of how subtle the reaction. The belief triggers the feeling that we are unsafe. The response is to need to be in control, so we are not relaxed and don't go with the flow. Our energies get into an activated state that stimulate the sympathetic nervous system. If we hold on to a certain belief system long enough, it will be triggered quite often and will result in a chronic "stressed-out" state of the body, ultimately resulting in physical disease.

First of all, the stress lowers the immune system, making us susceptible to outside pathogens. When the immune system is affected chronically, it can result in frequent infections, allergies, parasitic infestations, auto-immune conditions, and cancer.

Secondly, when a person is not relaxed and they are on guard, their breathing is affected. Rather than being slow and deep, stress makes breathing more rapid and shallow, preventing the lungs from properly filling. The lungs fill the blood with oxygen, which supplies nourishment to the tissues. In Chinese medicine, the lungs generate the Qi. This is another way of understanding how the Qi governs the blood and how the mind governs the Qi. When the mind is stressed, being resistant, and in control of the Qi, the lungs do not fill properly with air and the blood is therefore not nourished with oxygen, which leads to a poorly nourished body.

Thirdly, when someone uses his/her will to either be in control of situations or to stop the flow of their Qi (emotions), their muscles become chronically tight. Stress leads to tense muscles. When the muscles are tight, a person becomes rigid. Flow and flexibility promote health. Rigidity is synonymous with disease.

It is difficult to maintain perfect delineation of where everything starts and what is the cause of the imbalances and stress responses in the body. There is much overlap, with things affected simultaneously. For one, did the muscles become rigid because the rear-will chakras became controlling, which affected the flow of the front feeling chakra and made the person more sympathetic-active, which then increased the tension of the muscles? Or did the muscles tighten up because the person was uptight and was attempting to be controlling? It is all happening at the same time.

The important point to understand is that dis-ease starts in the mind. Since the Mind controls the Qi which controls the Blood, the stress has already become dis-ease right with the belief system that necessitates reality to be that way and not any way else (rigidity of mind). This gets carried down into the emotional level when the mind begins controlling the Qi through the chakras (rigidity of feeling). And then the blood and body are next to become fixated and dis-eased. The body is like a faithful dog responding to the commands of the mind. You say sit, it sits. You say roll over and play dead, it obeys.

> **Only the mind is capable of error. The body can act wrongly only when it is responding to misthought.**
> —*A Course in Miracles,*
> chapter 2, section IV, paragraph 2, verse 4.

The fact that the mind also resonates at a vibrational frequency that is much higher and much finer than the physical body in its material form also shows us that the body cannot be the cause of disease in the mind. Just as you cannot grab the light with your hand, or pick up gas molecules with large stones, the body does not directly influence the subtle energies of the mind. The mind can, however, observe the sick state of the body and become upset and disturbed, but this is a choice the person makes in the mind.

In his play, *Hamlet*, William Shakespeare wrote "There is nothing either good or bad, but thinking makes it so." And that is the truth. So in our practices, an excellent focus is to uncover what people need to believe that is making their reality right or wrong. Or we can determine what beliefs cause people to be controlling, judgmental, and stressed out. Here is the secret of treating the fundamental cause of disease in many, if not most, chronic diseases. And since people all believe different things about reality, the cure for their diseases lies in helping change their individual ways of thinking that stresses them out, causing their illness.

Even some chronic diseases that have resulted from environmental toxicity, or physical trauma, which seem to have an obvious source that is physical, can be rooted within the mind. In my clinic year, there was a woman visiting the clinic who had been paralyzed for many years from the waist down. Her story was that years ago, she was married to a man who physically abused her. One day, she decided that she was going to leave him. Upon telling him this, he became enraged and scared her so much that she backed off the balcony of the second floor of her house, fell and broke her back. For years she was paralyzed. She had tried many courses of treatment that yielded few results. Nothing would help her until she began to face the difficult feelings that she had toward her husband and even toward herself that she had suppressed. When she was able to face the past, and come to terms with the situation, she was able to move her legs again.

The healing power of Nature is always there to restore our bodies to health once we take our foot off the brakes in our internal energy systems. What is an obstacle to cure? Often, it is simply that the cause has not been removed and the dam that keeps back the healing power of Nature still holds strong. Perhaps even in the worst accidents that result in the most severe crippling and paralysis, there is still hope of treating the cause and restoring the person's mobility and health. It is only in how we limit Nature's ability to heal us that the healing power of Nature becomes limited.

In many cases that seem to require treating the physical symptoms, there is a root in the mental or emotional spheres that needs addressing. This is true in cases of idiopathic infertility, where the infertility has no apparent cause. Some infertile women deal successfully with the key mental and emotional issues that prevented them from conceiving. One such story concerned a woman who was terrified of having a handicapped child. She was so scared that she subconsciously refused to have a baby. She faced this issue, and understood her fear. She dealt with the possibility of having a handicapped child and found peace. She conceived soon after.

Another woman feared the responsibility of a child would diminish her own individuality. Even though she wanted a child, she had this very deep issue to deal with. She too prevented conception until she dealt with her fear.

Both of the women in these infertility cases, and in many others, could have undergone all the lab tests possible. Hormonal imbalances would not have been found. If they were, it still wouldn't matter. Attempting to correct the hormonal imbalance is not a way of working in harmony with Nature. There is nothing wrong with the woman's body. The body is simply reflecting what goes on in the mind. If the woman doesn't wish to have a child, it is a choice based in a very personal fear. The hormones act in accordance with the mind's choices. The same is true for a man with a low sperm count. His low sperm count is a reflection of some issue that he might have about being a man or a father. When his energy is freed from his issue, his testes will readily produce virile sperm and a healthy count.

These illustrations encourage us to become highly skilled at counseling and psychotherapy. This way, we can understand the patterns of belief system and judgmental thinking that cause disease in our copatients and can guide them to release these belief systems and judgments.

If people believe that other people cannot be trusted, their heart chakras will be affected, because it is the chakra through which we connect with others. People will use the negative intention from their belief system to control the will of the heart chakra to stop the flow of the heart. They don't want to feel the connection with others because they have deemed them as bad. Such people can become hard-hearted and unfeeling, because they do not trust others and view them as a threat. The heart can develop pathology like hardening of the coronary arteries, which is a reflection of the person's belief system. Their body in the surrounding area will also reflect what is going on in the mind. The muscles of their back around the third to the fifth thoracic area can become very tense which will influence the mobility of the spine. A chiropractor would examine the person and find fixations and subluxations in their spine, affecting the nerve plexus and causing a poor nourishment of the internal organs in that area. Adjustment of the thoracic vertebrae increases mobility in the area, which can liberate a lot of blocked energy and begin the healing process, but if the cause of the resistance and rigidity is not addressed, the person will continue to become tense in that area, creating fixations and subluxations, which will require frequent adjustments. This is often the case in chiropractic, because the cause is not being addressed in the person's mind.

If we examine this closely, we see that chiropractic medicine forces against where the body wishes to go. For example, let's imagine that the muscles are tense in the right thoracic area of T4 and are pulling that thoracic vertebra to the right (when examined with the copatient lying prone). This might be due to the person avoiding some pain in their heart, pulling away in their attempts to control the pain. Whatever the cause, there is tension in the muscles attached to T4, pulling it to the right. The chiropractic corrective measure would be to adjust T4 by pushing it forcedly and rapidly to the left, in the opposite direction from where it wants to go. This is forcing against the way the body wishes to go, in the same way that giving a hypotensive agent to combat high blood pressure does. It is, therefore, somewhat allopathic in nature.

When we contrast this way of treating the disharmony in the system with the way cranio-sacral therapy, osteopathy, homeopathy, and counseling work, we see the difference. These medicines work in harmony with nature by not forcing against the way the body, emotions, or the mind choose to go (in resistance and holding on to control pain and difficult issues).

In cranio-sacral therapy, the practitioner subtly detects the cranial rhythms of the body and feels the ways in which the energies attempt to flow. Just as in the way the rear chakras control the flow of energy, the energy of the person's system pushes against or fights to avoid something. If the flow of the energy needs to pull in a certain direction, the practitioner does not try to force it back in the other direction, but rather gently "encourages" the flow in that direction. We see the same philosophy at work in osteopathy, which incorporates cranio-sacral as part of its method of treatment. A person who has had an injury, for instance, whatever the level (spiritual, mental, emotional, physical), is brought through the ways in which the body has wound itself up escaping or running away from the injury. By going into the path the body has taken in response to an injury, the body unwinds itself and restores a lasting balance and healed response. The cranio-sacral therapist and osteopath therefore help reverse the process of resistance by first encouraging the very same direction of resistance. It is like the example of a ship moored to a dock. The captain wishes to set sail out to sea, so he/she lifts up the anchor. The ship is obviously stuck, and the rope taught with the tension of wishing to break free. The allopathic response to this would be either to cut the rope or empower the boat to push out to sea until the rope breaks or something else gives. Cranio-sacral and all therapies that work in harmony with Nature bring the ship closer to the dock to ease the tension on the rope, and then untie it.

Homeopathy also works in harmony with a person's mind, body, and spirit. If a person needs to dominate and be in control, he/she is given a substance in nature that affects the human being in the very same way when taken in a proving. If someone's muscles are tightly bunched up, the remedy they are given doesn't relax muscles, but tightens them in the very same fashion that the person is experiencing. Given something that tightens muscles in the same way they are already tightened works in this harmonious, untying-a-moored-ship fashion to reverse the whole tension process. If someone fears being enclosed in tight spaces or feels trapped in relationships, they are given a substance in nature that effects a healthy person to feel the very same way, so that they are brought into their fear and ultimately are able to see right through it.

In the movie K-PAX, Kevin Spacey's character, Prot, from the distant planet K-PAX, lets himself be admitted to a psychiatric hospital. During his stay, he helps teach people, including the doctors, some very beautiful lessons. Prot gives one of the patients, Howie, a task to strangle another patient, Ernie, who is terrified of suffocation and extremely paranoid of germs. When Ernie is revived after being suffocated, he is totally transformed and seems completely well. He says to the doctor;

> When I woke up, you know what I realized, Dr. Powell? Dying is something you have no control over. Why waste your life being afraid of it? I'll sleep on my stomach from now on. I'll eat fish with bones in it. I'll swallow the largest pill you can find. Bring it on! Ha ha. I feel good.

This act was homeopathically curative. Ernie was brought into his fears and realized they were no longer necessary. This is the secret of healing. I am uncertain whether the CNME would approve of our students learning the strangulation technique, but understanding this principle is of great importance in whole person medicine.

Counseling works to heal a person much in the same way that homeopathy does. This is especially true for the form of counseling and psychotherapy called Core Belief work. In this form of therapy, once the belief systems are discovered, the person goes into those beliefs and holds them in mind for a while. The belief system is "encouraged." By doing so, the person faces the source of their belief systems. We adopt belief systems to run from our pain, or from our feelings of insecurity and our fear of being out of control. By going into a belief system and holding on to it intentionally and voluntarily, the process reverses in the very same way—instead of holding on to the belief, the person willfully enters into the belief, ultimately reversing the resistance and control.

All forms of counseling have a profound effect on a person's health and well-being when the person comes face to face with their belief systems. When patients realize what they have been choosing to believe about themselves or reality and they make the decision to no longer think that way, healing begins. "I don't hold that as truth any longer. That is not what I choose to believe." The whole cascade of controlling Qi and controlling Blood that leads to disease begins to reverse itself once the control that comes from the source/core belief is released.

In all of these healing modalities that work in harmony with Nature, the healing process occurs because there is an acceptance of how the person tries to be. Then the body, emotions and mind can relax. It is the exact opposite of the original judgment and control that led to disease. A person has determined that something is bad (pain in the heart, feeling of being stupid) and so they fight against it, inwardly and outwardly. The healing process, therefore, must not be equally judgmental of the judgment and resistance in the system. That would involve burying it further beneath more judgment and would fulfill the universal truth that was stated above; "Everything in the Universe that is judged reacts by trying to prove it is worthy of existence." And so when the resistance is forced against, the person's energetic systems are going to take a stand to prove that their choice is fine. This happens in all realms of our being. If you try to get someone to see beyond his/her belief systems, he/she will cling to their notions of reality. Trying to make someone happy who is choosing to be sad by providing happy things to think about usually doesn't work because their choice is not being respected. Working in harmony with the healing power of Nature, all limiting choices that lead to disease and disharmony must therefore be respected and even given the space to remain the way they are. This promotes the healing process.

> **The curious paradox is that when I accept myself just as I am, then I can change.**
>
> —Carl Rogers

What this actually reveals to us is that disease is a messenger, a way of our body telling us that something is not in harmony. For this reason, illness is a gift to us, a way of deepening our relationships with ourselves. When we get sick, a messenger comes from a beautiful place to tap us on the shoulder and say, "There is something that you are not willing to see." We often get sick with minor colds and flus when we do not listen to our body's needs to rest and move at a pace that is more suited for our balance. Chronic disease is a manifestation of illness that has come about to teach us a life lesson, demonstrating the ways in which we have chosen to live in opposition to Mother Nature and with all of creation. In approaching illness with this philosophy, it becomes a sacred realm where kernels of truth await us. It becomes an opportunity for us to learn, grow, and reconnect with the beauty of life all around us. In healing ourselves at the root of chronic illness, in the whole of who we are, we become healthy and aware in a way that far surpasses our state of being as we were before we got sick.

The allopathic approach does not respect this process. It regards illness as something that must be wiped out, pushed against and buried. When there is no acceptance of the disease we have chosen or manifested, there is no way to learn these lessons and to grow as people, deepening our connection with Nature. Even if we learn to perfectly control disease, people will not mature in relation to themselves and will remain unwise. The world will continue to be filled with people who do not understand the deeper connections to Nature. Such people will continue to find it easy to do things like pollute, destroy forests and other natural habitats, and other actions that reflect the war on Nature they have within themselves. Therefore it is not solely through the treatment of sick people that we fulfill our purpose to humanity. Through shedding the proper light on the whole process of disease, how and why it manifests, we can dispel the fear that governs medicine. We can empower people to think properly about their health, by understanding their mind-body connection, and to become more whole people in response to the holism of our medicine.

The Mosquito Meditation

Aka "The Acupuncture of Nature Meditation,"
"Mastering Psora Meditation"

This is quite a fun meditation that demonstrates how Mother Nature is always seeking our best interest. The purpose of this meditation is to heal and rekindle a trust in Nature.

Our skin has a surface energy that is supplied by the acupuncture meridians. At the acupuncture points, there is a small electro-magnetic charge that creates a surface tension. Where the acupuncture point or meridian is blocked or deficient, the surface tension will be compromised. Amazingly, mosquitoes will only bite you in the place where your energy is blocked. In fact, I believe they are unable to penetrate your skin to feed on your blood in an area that is energetically balanced and healthy because the surface tension repels them.

Here is how the meditation goes:

Sit in an area that has mosquitoes. It is recommended you choose an area without too many mosquitoes at first, or it can be overwhelming. You will notice that the mosquitoes try to land on your body and will not bite you in the areas where your skin's electrical potential is healthy and in good integrity. They will bite you where your energy is blocked. Relax as deeply as possible and open yourself up to *allow* the mosquitoes to find the points of blockage. Tune in to Nature and allow the mosquitoes to land on you and to bite you where they choose. Each time a mosquito swoops down onto your skin, say "Thank you, Mrs. Mosquito." (Only the females feed). You will observe that when you allow them total and complete access to your skin without holding back or being afraid, they will only rarely bite. This is a sign that you are in harmony with Nature. They will bounce around until they find a place of blockage. And when they do bite you, it is Mother Nature performing acupuncture on you. Unfortunately, mosquitoes often don't know when to stop.

So gently brush them off your skin after they have bitten you for 20–30 seconds.

Here is another challenge of this exercise—Once the mosquitoes do bite you, you must not scratch at all. Allow the itch to go as deeply as it can. The venom of the mosquitoes is causing a healthy healing reaction. By not scratching, you are confronting Psora, the oldest miasm that has affected the human being the longest, which is sometimes referred to as "Suppressed itch." Allowing the itch to continue without scratching or suppressing it, is the most healing part of this meditation and is what confronts Psora. When someone sits passively in an area of many mosquitoes without any artificial or natural substances on his/her body (to drive away mosquitoes) and he/she has not ingested inordinate amounts of vitamin B1, and the mosquitoes don't bite at all, that person has become a Psora Master.

CHAPTER 4

Allopathic and Naturopathic:
Finding the Balance

THE DISCUSSIONS OF THIS BOOK reveal the importance of establishing the foundation of naturopathic medicine, in our philosophy, rooted in Mother Nature. In order to ensure this, we must be very clear that there is a great purpose behind realigning the education with the roots that serve the profession and all people who will be touched by naturopathic medicine. To ensure that naturopaths feel comfortable practicing the pure form of our medicine freely in the world, we do require a certain detachment from political correctness that has gone slightly overboard. It is simply not serving us in bringing naturopathic medicine to the public.

We all know political correctness (PC). People become politically correct in attempts to balance negative situations where people have been treated unfairly. In response to racism, sexism, and injustice, this is great. If there were events in the Olympics for athletes to demonstrate their prowess in political correctness, Naturopathic medicine would get the gold. The prize-winning team would consist of naturopathic doctors and students highly skilled in political correctness. More than any other profession, naturopathic medicine is politically correct. With its ranks filled with healers, activists, New Agers and people of all sexual orientations, it is on the cutting edge of non-judgmentalness and PC. But the naturopathic team would have to be careful not to go overboard into political over-correctness in the event of toe stepping, where they might be tempted to apologize when someone stepped on their own toes. We must be equally cautious not to apologize for practicing naturopathic medicine in the way it was conceived.

When a person has an apologetic attitude, people don't take them seriously and often walk all over them. The hesitant, apologetic attitude is inadvertently and often subconsciously a way of admitting that he/she thinks there is something wrong with him/herself. Otherwise, why be so apologetic? This is often seen in naturopathic medicine, in clinics where practitioners hesitate and apologize to lead their copatients down the healing path. The attitude is often accompanied by a feeling that we are doing something wrong by being who we are. This has to do with the fear of being censured and labeled as a witch, practicing medicine in a way that is outside of the box, because the fear is not seen when naturopaths practice green (natural) allopathy because it is already established and accepted. It is time for naturopaths to stand up bravely and to trust in the validity and efficacy of our medicine as it is practiced in harmony with the healing power of Nature, even in those ways that are not currently accepted by the establishment of science.

I have often seen naturopaths bravely giving talks and seminars if they feel they have enough scientific evidence to support their treatment protocols. The protocols that are presented are often allopathic in nature and therefore, have a proven basis that is easy to lean on. We can be equally brave in explaining whole person medicine, the mind-body connection, and how each person is responsible for his/her own health. To do so, it is time to come out of the cocoon where the profession has been metamorphosing, and shed our hesitancy and apologetic attitude for being a young profession with something new and special to offer the world.

Political correctness can also go overboard in situations where important decisions must be made for the future of the profession. Yet, everyone accepts differences in opinion that lead the profession in different directions. How do you affect change with such an attitude? Overly PC stunts the growth of arguments that can lead to change and resolution of disharmonies when there exists opposing points of view. Everyone being entitled to one's opinion is healthy PC. But when there are opinions that lead the profession in opposite directions and they are allowed to coexist without resolution, this is POC (Political over-correctness).

Many have said that our profession, being comprised of so many strong-minded and strong-willed people, will naturally be divided between differing opinions. I am the first to agree with that IF it is within the realm of where the roots of our philosophy are being taught and practiced. Naturally, there are countless different ways of practicing our medicine because it is undefined, with each unique copatient, by each unique naturopath. We begin to enter in POC territory when people claim that the profession being divided *in philosophy* between the allopathic model and the naturopathic healing paradigm is okay. Here we need to provide some clear delineation. The delineation is not for the purpose of regulating naturopaths who are already out in the field practicing as they wish, often as a product of their education. The purpose of the delineation is to ensure that the education gets properly aligned with the way of naturopathic medicine as defined by our philosophy. It is essential that we establish the overall foundation of our medicine upon the roots of Mother Nature, where the healing way of whole person naturopathy becomes the standard.

If we do not properly root our profession and education in our philosophy, POC becomes harmful to the profession, as it would to any profession or organization that is based upon principles and then accepts when those principles are not being embraced and carried forward.

It is not POC that causes the division within our ranks and education. It simply allows it to continue. Perhaps, being a healing profession that has not entirely established itself as credible amongst the public, it is the fear of judgment and censorship that divides our ranks the most. As within any individual who lives concerned about what the world thinks, he/she will be split between the true nature, and the desire to prove him/herself, which is not a natural process. Whatever the case may be, we must overcome our overly politically correct tendencies to ensure that we align our profession in the right direction. We do this not just for ourselves but for each and every person we will come to influence, through our direct one-on-one consultations, to our influence through the media, education, the healthcare system and the government. We must get together as one to serve humanity with the skills and gifts we have to share.

Being true to our medicine does not mean that the allopathic approach plays no role in naturopathy or in the world. It is important to understand the situations in which the allopathic and conventional approaches are still valid. However, the balance that must be met is not a 1:1 ratio. Once our roots are firmly re-established, we will naturally have room to teach allopathic protocols for cases and situations requiring symptom and disease-based treatment. And these protocols will be taught in a clear way that indicates to students that they are learning allopathic measures for *special* cases that require such protocols, not mixed in and indiscernible from the rest of the program.

Naturopathic medicine has established a wide range of protocols for the allopathic treatment of disease and its symptoms using natural products, herbs, and non-toxic supplements. This is also a gift to the world, yet it is not something that our profession should become particularly attached to, or focus too much attention on, since it is quite easy for medical doctors also to practice allopathic medicine using natural supplements. In fact, this is already occurring today. More and more doctors, and the pharmaceutical industry, are adopting and suggesting natural supplements. In the near future, if the foundation of naturopathic medicine were still allopathic, our profession would become swallowed up and out-competed by medical doctors, who are the experts of allopathic medicine. Medical doctors are better skilled and better equipped at diagnosing and treating disease. They are disease experts.

Many people also go to health food stores to find their own supplemental, vitamin and herbal solutions to their ailments. The Internet is a sea of information for people to learn abundant information about natural therapies and supplements to treat themselves allopathically. If we play in the allopathic field, we will become obsolete and redundant. What slice of the allopathic pie would naturopathic medicine have left? Who would want to pay hundreds of dollars to go see a naturopath when he/she can go to a medical doctor and be covered by Medicare and insurance or simply use health food stores and the Internet to find their own solution?

It is in the roots of whole person naturopathy, in a totally different and newfound territory, where our profession is really needed. It is in helping the world adapt to Nature's path and not adapting to the way of conventional medicine that our profession stands a chance of surviving. Not only will we survive, but rather we will thrive and be joyous in fulfilling our doctor-as-teacher role to humanity by helping shift from the allopathic paradigm of treating the symptoms of disease, to the healing paradigm.

There are certain cases that will still require allopathic treatment. We will call these "Exceptional cases." An example of an exceptional case is when copatients are near death and have no vital energy to heal themselves. In such cases, they are completely taken out of the picture of their own health because they are so weak and have no vitality or strength to be brought through the healing process. Even giving homeopathic remedies during such times will provide little to no improvement. Therefore, it is necessary to give them support through supplementation, or treat them symptomatically and allopathically in order to save their lives. Often the elderly require allopathic treatment when they are very old and so attached to the way of thinking of their younger days that it is beyond their abilities to open up and share their issues.

Sometimes people are too afraid to let go of their belief systems, fear and control patterns. They are also petrified of their disease in general. At such times, the combination of fear of their healing process and of their disease calls for giving the person something from the outside to provide a sense of security. Such a treatment isn't going to cure them, because we understand that through treating the cause and the whole person that a cure is brought forth. But it will help them lean on a crutch until they feel capable of either subconsciously or consciously facing the cause of their illness and taking responsibility for their health.

Conventional medicine will always have a role in society. Even when people take responsibility for their health and undergo whole person healing, conventional medicine will still play a role in emergency and traumatic situations, cases that are near-death, cases that require surgery to set bones and fix destroyed joints, and to transplant or fix non-functioning organs. In the future, medical advances will be able to increase longevity by improving the technology in areas of organ transplantation, surgery, end-stage cancer, and other aggressive, life-threatening diseases.

Other Exceptional cases can involve injury, where something is knocked out of place and is stuck. Osteopathy can help a person go into a lesion from trauma when the vertebra is on its normal plane of rotation. If a vertebra gets knocked off of its normal plane of rotation, due to one or several injuries, it has little chance of correcting itself and must be forced back into place. Sometimes hemorrhoids can "pop out" from straining at stool or during pregnancy. A whole person, unique approach is indicated to increase a person's vitality and deal with the cause of weakness that led to the hemorrhoids, which will reverse the process. Other times, the hemorrhoids must be dealt with directly because they are hanging out of place and cannot be retracted. Ideally, when you turn up the healing power of Nature in a person's body by removing the dams of resistance (causes of disease) that ebb its flow, *anything* and *everything* can heal. Even in a case of a vertebra out of alignment, the innate intelligence of the body knows how to correct it. When a weakened area with hemorrhoids is suffused with healing Qi, the body will correct itself by slowly contracting and retracting the hemorrhoids. But not all cases can be treated with the pure form of our medicine, and the ideal, for whatever reason, might be inaccessible. So we have the capacity to refer or treat allopathically.

Naturopaths will always have to be able to recognize when it is time to refer a copatient to conventional medicine or when to treat the case allopathically. There is no real way to define when that needs to be. It is determined by the state of the copatient, his/her decision of how to be treated, as well as by the confidence and experience of the naturopath.

In the HOA on pg. 42, it is written that the core curriculum must prepare students to, "Provide health care that holds to each patient's best interest." This of course means that the copatient's decision is always ultimate. Yet copatients do not always know what is in their best interest when dealing with their health, especially if they have been raised in the allopathic paradigm. Since we are Nature doctors, we understand that the best interest for copatients lies in dealing with their issues and the causes of their diseases in their roots, while taking responsibility for their own health. If copatients prefer simply to have their symptoms or disease dealt with, is it in their best interest to just treat their constipation, migraines, or back pain without addressing the rest? No. Allopathic treatment, when the case does not require it, is not in the copatient's best interest. People have gotten lazy and do not understand the connection between how they choose to live and their health. They want a quick fix. It is in their best interest that the naturopathic doctor makes every effort to help them understand the mind-body connection, how the process of disease develops, and how it can be reversed. Here it is essential not to be POC, rather to be clear on what is important, in a firm and gentle manner.

As a naturopath's skills increase in whole person medicine, and people are willing to deal with their issues in a holistic fashion, the number of cases requiring allopathic or conventional treatment will decrease. More and more chronic cases of disease will walk down the path of healing, where a person not only gets better physically and emotionally, but their entire outlook on, and relationship with, life improves.

As primary health care providers we have the capacity to treat the whole person and teach the principles of healthy living, unaffected by any other models of medicine. We have the opportunity also to educate people in the knowledge that they are in charge of their own health. Cases in which naturopath and medical doctor work together can benefit the copatient when necessary, as in Exceptional cases. When we work with medical doctors, the allopathic approach usually presides. It must. If we were to try to treat holistically and at the cause during allopathic treatment, it would confuse the patients, being led in one direction to heal from within and at the cause, and also being led in the other direction by having their symptoms palliated and treated. Because of the nature of allopathic treatment, whole person healing does not work nearly as well and we must then act as complement, providing the patients with support while they go through the allopathic process. That is okay.

Having unopposed freedom in a case helps empower copatients to make changes in their lives and see the effectiveness of whole person healing. That is our goal. This is in the copatient's best interest. This gives us the conviction to be clear, firm, and to release political overcorrectness. That is part of finding the balance between knowing when to treat allopathically or refer to conventional medicine, and when to help a person heal solely through holistic means. As our profession emerges, our practitioners will find fewer and fewer cases that require allopathic palliation of disease.

When this shift occurs in our education, new students who would have ordinarily sat on the fence and been steered whatever way the curriculum showed them, will be proud to embrace the healing paradigm. Students debating whether to go into conventional medicine or naturopathic medicine will find it easier to trust the path less taken when they see the shift amongst the supervisors and teachers of the colleges and the professionals in the field. Then, with trust and conviction of the efficacy and validity of our medicine, it will become the path most taken and the accepted medicine of the time.

This conviction has to start with each of us now stepping out of the politically over-correct world, where students demand the curriculum provide them with what they need to be whole NDs, and where naturopaths who know the model of healing are placed in teaching positions and positions of administration. The colleges are the anchors of our profession, the spawning grounds of the colony of naturopathic medicine. Get the education right and aligned with its purpose, and it will positively impact the growth of our healing doctors. In order to make change, you have to be very clear and firm about what needs to change. This means you must not be overboard with political correctness or else nothing will get done, or you will accept situations not in the copatient's best interest. If everything is okay now in our profession and the world of medicine as it is, what needs to change?

A lot.

CHAPTER 5

Diagnosis and Prognosis

DIAGNOSIS AND PROGNOSIS are two terms that we will use less and less in our medicine. These terms create a box within which patients are squeezed. When we feel the need to use diagnosis and prognosis in our practices, we treat disease, not individuals. In some cases, it doesn't hurt to know the medical diagnosis of a copatient's condition, such as for acute conditions where it is necessary to treat the symptoms to provide relief. But in chronic disease, diagnosis and prognosis do not serve you to treat naturopathically along the lines of our philosophy.

The very notion of labeling disease is a limiting concept. With the label of a disease comes a range of symptoms and ideas that puts everyone with that disease under the same umbrella. If we, as naturopaths, are to treat each person as an individual, it requires us to see that each person's experience of disease is entirely personal, subjective, and unique. Thus, to study diseases the way we have observed them medically is absurd because you are not treating disease, but individuals. You treat people, on all their levels—in their diets (physical), their belief systems and fears (mental), their pain and sufferings (emotional) and their connection with the Universe (spiritual). Whatever the disease, whatever the diagnosis, has no bearing on your course of action as a naturopath. The temptation to treat allopathically is there, especially for someone new to practice. If you are handed a diagnosis or determine one on your own, it further increases the likelihood of using that definition of disease to treat the disease and not the whole person. It also becomes an obstacle if you or the copatient have become enmeshed in the whole belief and idea about that disease.

In this light, prognosis is also something that naturopaths must avoid. Why? Because all the prognoses that we study come from the observation of diseases treated according to the allopathic way—mechanistically, symptomatically, and often impersonally, without a deep connection to the copatient. If whole person naturopathic medicine or other healing medicines had been the key players, for the last century or two, treating whole individuals in harmony with nature, the prognoses of diseases would be very, very different. Actually, we might not even have a section in our textbooks about the prognosis of disease because we would understand that it depends on the individuals, on their attitudes, their willingness to take responsibility for their health, their relationships with themselves and their practitioners, and not on the disease. Imagine how much we have severed ourselves from our own power to heal and influenced our health by creating such delineating definitions from the diagnosis and prognosis of disease? Where is the individual in that? If our governments continued not to allow naturopaths to diagnose, it would be a blessing, because we wouldn't fall so often into the temptation of unnecessarily treating the disease.

Prognosis is a word that should be wiped out of our vocabulary. Eventually, the term "diagnosis" will be given less and less importance, but it is a larger leap to make, and does sometimes serve a purpose in acute illness and allopathic treatment.

Another reason why we must understand the necessity of releasing the emphasis on diagnosis and prognosis in naturopathic medicine is because of the negative effects these approaches to medicine have on the patient. This negative effect is called the "nocebo" effect. The placebo effect is the positive and often beneficial effect on a patient's health caused by the doctor's declarations and enthusiasm about the outcome of disease. "Take this, it's really gonna help." This power that patients have given doctors must be cleared, but it still exists, so the picture that all doctors paint for their patients and copatients, has a huge effect. "You're going to do just fine." Wow!

Thanks, Doc. Sigh of Relief. Patients shouldn't take every word that comes out of a doctor's mouth as the gospel truth. We have to help them understand this.

Unfortunately, the nocebo effect is the other end of the spectrum from the placebo effect's positive influence on our health. "This is a very serious condition you have. You only have a few months to live." Oh no! I only have a few months to live. Imagine being told that and believing it?!!? How can doctors make such declarations when there are stories of miracles that occur when people fight until the end! This is really playing God in a way that might be considered criminal at some point in our future.

The diagnosis and subsequent prognosis of cancer is something that is teeming with the nocebo effect. There are many anecdotes about people going to their doctor because they bumped their knee or for something completely benign and the doctor haphazardly discovers a cancer that has been latent in the person. Sometimes these undiagnosed cancers have existed in the person for decades. Undoubtedly the cancer has had some effect on their health, but they have continued to live without too much trouble until they are told they have cancer. Then they die shortly afterwards.

When I was diagnosed in 1995 with Myasthenia Gravis, I learned about the prognosis of that disease and what it meant for a person's life. Very bleak indeed. The disease was said to be progressive, slowly worsening, and that there was no cure. I was told that I would have to at least be on Mestinon (acetylcholine-esterase inhibitor) for the rest of my life. I was told that might not be enough as it often didn't work for many people, and so I'd have to consider Prednisone. Prednisone doesn't work for everyone either. Another course of action that many patients of Myasthenia Gravis (M.G.) end up following is thymectomy—the complete removal of the thymus gland. This too works for some, and not for others. I was told that if the disease continued to progress with the symptoms of muscular paralysis or weakness, there was always the other option of weekly blood transfusions.

Imagine all the people who place all the power for their health in the hands of this diagnosis and prognosis? It is progressive and incurable. The aura that surrounds M.G. is bleak and people with the disease become hopelessly shackled to it. They live in wheelchairs, so weak they cannot do a thing on their own, and some eventually die.

Lou Klein, a Canadian homeopath, has cured several cases of M.G. with homeopathy. If one person can be cured, just one, it punches a hole in the belief system about the prognosis of the disease that MUST show all others with that disease the *potential* for cure. And I am certain that for *every* disease out there, there has been at least one person who has cured themselves or been cured. Those people with the symptoms of muscular weakness that we have called Myasthenia Gravis who put their power into the diagnosis are subject to a poor prognosis. Yet how can any person who has heard of a cure, even one, continue to say that the disease is incurable?

Thank goodness I never believed in the diagnosis and prognosis or else I, too, might be paralyzed in a wheelchair today, or even dead. It has been through the examination of myself on all levels of my being, through remembering to be true to myself, through taking the power of health into my own hands, and knowing that I *could* heal myself, that I have continued to live since 1995 with Myasthenia Gravis without any allopathic medical intervention. Even though some symptoms remain, I have not been stopped for one day from participating in activities that I have always loved, like playing soccer, golf, hockey, and practicing Karate.

We naturopathic doctors are so needed in this world to show the way outside of the boxes of disease-based treatment and all the confinements of the beliefs surrounding diagnosis and prognosis. In simply providing people with the hope to understand that there is no such thing as prognosis of disease because each person is different and the healing power of Nature is available to all who put their trust and energy into it, we can really help people. We are dealing with people's lives. There is no reason we should associate with ideas of diagnosis and prognosis when they do not provide a positive potential, especially when people being cured through healing means have destroyed the certainty of a disease ending poorly.

Like the man, Roger Bannister, who ran the four-minute mile and showed everyone it could be done, no longer could people state that it could not be done. And naturopaths should no longer live within the confinements of prognosis and diagnosis.

In any case, you assess the prognosis of diseases by how the copatient feels, by their levels of energy, their mood, their sexual desire, their joie de vivre. You measure it by the shine in their eyes, their presence, the movement of their bowels. You assess it on all levels. Even when some of the symptoms of their so-called disease persist, but the copatients feel happy, stronger, more alive, they are improving.

Naturopathic prognosis should state that when people go to see a naturopath who works in harmony with Nature and naturopathic philosophy, their health will improve as soon as the first visit begins, regardless of the disease. This is a good notion and not unrealistic. Even in cases of cancer, if you begin to work with diet, and you help the copatients improve their relationships with themselves and their loved ones, the harmful patterns of living that caused their bodies to break down into cancer will reverse themselves. Perhaps this change will not show itself instantly in the size of a tumour or on its markers, but the negative energies of disharmony, being reversed and cleared, will no longer continue to bring that person towards death, and the physical manifestations of the cancer will slowly improve. We must also remember that if they do die, they might have chosen to die and we can only be with them during their passing. No medicine in heaven or on earth could bring such people back if in their hearts they have chosen to leave us, or however Mother Nature decides these things. We do not have the responsibility, nor the capacity, to understand the final outcome of anyone's life.

The power that diagnosis and prognosis have over our health, and the potential to elicit the nocebo effect, is harmful and negative.

It is a power that no doctor should possess, N.D. or M.D.. When our copatients understand fully and completely their power and responsibility for their health, it will then not be possible for their health to decline just because they are told it will, unless, of course, they choose to believe it. Understanding that, we should dissociate ourselves from these two medical terms in our education and in our practices. By doing that, we can bring great amounts of healing to people from the free-flowing power of Nature and establish a completely different understanding of the potential for cure outside of the defined boxes of disease and its prognosis.

CHAPTER 6

Malpractice:
Dispelling the Fear for the Naturopaths

ONE OF THE GREATEST PROBLEMS that medical doctors face is malpractice. Malpractice insurance is incredibly costly because of all the times doctors are sued for malpractice. This fear of malpractice lawsuit also overshadows the naturopathic profession. Yet this is not a worry that is necessary for naturopathic doctors. When one is worried or afraid, one's every move is influenced negatively. It is not only for this reason that we should not spend any of our time worrying about being sued, but in understanding that the same conditions that lead medical doctors to get sued do not apply to us when we are practicing naturopathic medicine in accordance with our philosophy.

There are several problems with conventional medicine that set up doctors to get sued. First of all, medical doctors take total and complete responsibility for people's health. Conventional medicine makes declarations of how people will feel, how they should or shouldn't feel, and how much time they have to live. People are often discouraged to seek their own solutions to their health. Medical doctors diagnose and treat disease without involving the patient at all. Patients are given a drug, or surgery is performed upon them and the patient is the passive observer. This kind of medicine has been called, "Playing God." And it is, because it takes away the power a person has to heal themselves and to make decisions about their own health. If medical doctors didn't try to be God in the realm of our health, but rather facilitators and guides, as they could be, people wouldn't take such aggressive action against them when they make a mistake. But it is not uncommon for doctors to get angry with people for thinking that they could possibly know what is influencing their health, or for thinking they have an idea as to how to help themselves. This is not true for every doctor, but there is a majority who believe they have the monopoly over our health. Because of this belief amongst MDs and the idea that they carry all the answers, when they make a mistake, their patients become angry and disappointed. Some of these patients will want to sue. When naturopathic doctors act as teachers to encourage people to take responsibility for their own health, the threat of malpractice is dissipated.

People who are responsible for their own health and understand how empowering it is, do not consider lawsuits. If people come to us and offer us all the eggs of their health to carry in one basket, we will decline. Not because we are afraid of the responsibility. By helping people understand how they are in charge of their own health, and not only that, but that they are capable of healing themselves (even without anyone else's help), they appreciate you. You have given them something, not taken anything away.

The goal of the naturopath is to become obsolete
—Anonymous

That is our goal globally and in each individual case: to help people be totally well and to give them the necessary tools to be so healthy that they never have to visit us again. What a strange sort of profession that sets itself up to be ultimately unnecessary! That is how special we are. Imagine an industry that doesn't work in this way but profits from disease... think about it.

It is also true to say that we don't make people sick, so we are also not *responsible* for getting them better. The power and responsibility lie within the individual, with the copatient. When you focus on the positive implications of this, you will see that in such a medicine where people understand their own responsibility, there is no fear of people suing you, because they did not give you the power in the first place to make or break their health, nor did you accept it. Remember this. It is an essential part of practicing within the healing paradigm. In healing, you recognize the truth that all the healing power of Nature comes about through the individual, in the individual from Nature. The healing isn't coming from you. You're simply assisting. Give the credit to your copatients. They will be grateful that they're feeling better and grateful to you. That is really all that matters. Again, what a strange profession that offers its services without taking credit for any of its successes. Well, of course you can, but you also cannot. And if you do start to take responsibility for the healing you will begin to interfere with the copatient's own power to heal themselves. We healers often do this because we want to help people heal so much that we forget the universal law of personal empowerment. In other cases, it makes us feel better to take responsibility for the cure.

At this point, we do not have the devices sensitive enough to determine a person's deepest choice of whether or not to stay on this earth. We also cannot detect with our sensors and tools if God/the Great Spirit/Mother Nature has not reached down to claim a person back to the Source. When people who are very ill and close to death choose to work with you on their health and they understand their responsibility, there is a truly beautiful energy and force working between you and them that burns brightly. They know you are not responsible for their life or death. And when you know and trust in that as well, you are free to help the person as much as possible. And who knows? You may even bring forth a miracle.

Whatever it is that determines how one person will live and another person will die, whether it is their own fighting will, or God's will, or chance, it is not your responsibility. So don't worry about it. If you do worry, you will simply taint with fear the purity of your connection with your copatient. Fear is the source of so much disease and need not exist in your practice.

Of course, don't go to the opposite extreme and start saying "You didn't get better, it's not my fault, you just didn't take responsibility." The truth is that the healing comes from within the copatient, but your aide and the remedies that you select, the counseling you do, or the points you needle, are definitely going to help make a difference when they are well selected. That is where your skill is necessary and your art and science essential. That is why we're there, not to take control over people's health, but to help people get better. If you choose a remedy and nothing happens, or you needle and there is no reaction, don't say that you are not responsible for your copatient's health, to blame *them* for not taking responsibility for their own health just because your treatment did nothing. That is absurd. Even though we are asked to give up responsibility over a copatient's health, we still need to be as present and involved as we can be in each and every case.

Another of the fears that I have seen naturopaths express is the fear of missing a diagnosis and the resultant repercussions—an aneurysm, a septic appendix, or a brain tumour. This again is the fear that a doctor has of failing to save a person's life. It comes from the general idea that a patient's life is in your hands. This is an incorrect way of thinking in practice of medicine, especially naturopathic medicine, that is not truthful. If you believe you have the responsibility for a person's life and you miss something, then you are responsible. But you are not responsible. You didn't get them sick, so you are not responsible for getting them better. The whole relationship that the general public has had with the medical profession hasn't been in balance because people wait until they are so sick that they require serious and sometimes heroic measures to save their lives. Why do they wait? Because they take no responsibility for their health. It is at the point when they are so broken down that they turn to the medical profession to make it better. This relationship is unhealthy, because it doesn't work well for doctors and patients and it is not truthful in the first place. As naturopaths, this relationship must be corrected to establish the responsibility for a copatient's health in the proper place; their own hands. Therefore, as primary health care physicians, we must not work with the intention that if we miss diagnoses that can result in serious illness or even death, that we are responsible. If those people did not go to see a doctor, they could still have been very sick or died. In other words, "Do no harm," does not encompass saving people from dying, or saving them from the disease they have already manifested in their body. "Do no harm" means that your medical intervention should cause no harm in a person, which is something that will never happen when you are working in harmony with the healing power of Nature. If someone comes into your office with a rigid abdomen and pain referring to the umbilicus and you don't diagnose acute appendicitis, *have you done any harm*? No. Unless you believe you are responsible for your copatient's health. The fear surrounding medicine is so strong because the thinking has forgotten this fundamental truth about our health; the responsibility lies with the copatient. And if people still do not wish to become aware of how their lifestyle and consciousness affect their health, that remains their choice.

Removing ourselves from the responsibility for copatients' lives and health is one of the greater hurdles in setting naturopathic medicine in a pure place. You have to take the time to see through the fear and see the harmony with Nature in giving responsibility back where it counts. In helping people make a switch from allopathic primary health care to naturopathic primary health care, our role is not to give them more of the same, but to give something new. This is one of the major factors that makes our naturopathic curriculum into something it is not.

Of course in caring for our copatients, we do everything we can to assure their safety along with their health. By releasing the fear of missing diagnoses, we are not saying that we wish to pretend that something is okay when it is not. We don't want to see perfect health when there is illness. If we suspect that a copatient is seriously ill, sending him/her to the emergency room is always an important option. In fact, conventional medicine will continue to play that role—the treatment of acute and threatening illness or trauma that place a person's life at risk.

Another reason that medicine can predispose the physician towards malpractice lawsuits is when it is aggressive and invasive. When a naturopath gives a homeopathic remedy, or suggests a change from wheat to spelt or kamut, he/she is not at risk of removing the wrong kidney, or severing a nerve during surgery. Counseling, homeopathy, nutrition, hydrotherapy, flower remedies, massage, cranio-sacral therapy, and hands-on-healing are all wonderful techniques that not only help people feel healthier and more well-balanced, but are also incredibly gentle. When the naturopath guides patients deeper into their own understanding of themselves, they do not run the risk of overwhelming the patient with too many toxic drugs, nor of causing many harmful, iatrogenic effects. True, conventional medicine is less barbaric and invasive today than it used to be, where drilling holes in peoples' heads to relieve them of headaches, or bleeding people to remove toxicity was considered normal practice. In relation to our naturopathic paradigm with the lasting healing effects of our gentle, non-invasive medicine, we do see that conventional medicine still removes organs that are sick and under-functioning when it is unnecessary, and still treats disease as if it is something that has to be eradicated from the body. These aggressive, invasive approaches to healthcare increase the risk of error and damage, iatrogenesis and adverse effects that then increase the risk in the profession of malpractice and lawsuit.

Naturopathy, practiced in harmony with the healing power of nature and not fighting against it, does not run the risk of injuring people or causing adverse effects. In addition to that, naturopaths take the time to get to know people on all their levels. Our history and case-taking often takes over an hour, sometimes two hours.

People who are listened to for hours, who develop a heart-felt relationship with their healers, do not think of suing. Naturopaths take a good case history, involving all levels of their copatients' being. As the relationship between naturopath and copatient develops, the naturopath will probably know more about that person, in all realms of their lives, than any other person. There is an exchange of trust between physician and copatient, something that is often missing in conventional medicine. Such a relationship does not walk down the road of malpractice. The relationships, therefore, between medical doctor and patient often remain impersonal, which facilitates patients taking legal action against their doctors whom they feel do not care about them.

Having personal relationships of great care and understanding, teaching copatients to take responsibility for their own health, and using gentle, non-invasive medicines that work in harmony with nature and do not force against the body's natural tendency to heal, naturopathic doctors are at no risk of being sued. So we see that we need not over concern ourselves, nor gear our education around avoiding things that may get us sued. I would encourage practitioners not to take malpractice insurance. The whole energy surrounding it is faulty in thinking, fear-based and only interferes with the healing process. When you associate so closely with something that is outside of yourself, you begin to adopt its way of thinking. By dissociating ourselves from the beliefs of established science and medicine and the need to be recognized as credible within that paradigm, we dissociate from the fears and worries that go hand in hand with that model of thinking. Then, rather than expending so much time trying to avoid mistakes, we can practice our joyous medicine freely and liberate a lot of time and energy in our education to be devoted to studies and courses that build us into who we are.

CHAPTER 7

The Different Practitioners and Modalities:
Allopathic or Healing Paradigm?

ANY ONE OF THE MODALITIES that we use (herbal medicine, homeopathy, acupuncture, nutrition, etc.) can be applied holistically to treat the whole person or applied allopathically to treat symptoms and disease. Even counseling can be used allopathically, simply by telling the copatient what they need to do. It is quite easy to employ herbal medicine allopathically because we have studied the actions of its constituents and we know which herbs will be beneficial in which disease or how they will affect the physical body. Nutritional supplementation is also often used in a palliative fashion, not to treat the root or the whole person, but to treat the disease and its symptoms. Even two of the more healing methods which have the capacity to treat all levels of the human being, homeopathy and acupuncture, can be used to treat symptoms. Thus it is the intention, not the modality itself, which dictates whether we employ the use of our medicine in an allopathic fashion or in a way that is aligned with naturopathic medicine. And in treating naturopathically, we benefit our copatients much more than if we simply use the modalities of our medicine allopathically. Treated holistically, copatients' health improves hand in hand with the betterment of their lives, their views of reality and how they feel about themselves.

In my awareness, there are three ways of practicing naturopathy. One of these is not holistic, but allopathic in nature. It is the way of the "green M.D." It is the use of all the modalities of our medicine to treat the symptoms of disease. It is good for a naturopath to have knowledge and skills in order to know how to do this when necessary, but when it is used in the majority of the time, especially in the treatment of chronic disease, the essence of the medicine is not being practiced.

Those medical doctors who employ some of the tools we use and use herbs and organic supplements to treat disease are taking their medicine to a better, less toxic place. So let them. If they make their treatments less invasive and safer, we can even help them towards doing that in the best way, through educational seminars and through literature. Our understanding of herbal medicine and supplementation can facilitate their growth in the alternative direction. But if we do the same, if a large number of our practitioners are simply practicing the way of the allopath, the green M.D., with our different modalities, then we are not fulfilling the principles of our philosophy. We also run the risk of being overpowered by the part of conventional medicine that is becoming more "green." What is going to set us apart if we treat allopathically with our natural modalities as they do?

Another way of practicing is to work in harmony with our philosophy and employ the use of the different modalities of healing; namely homeopathy, traditional Chinese medicine, herbal medicine, nutrition, counseling, and hydrotherapy. We can also employ other techniques that are not part of the program such as cranio-sacral therapy, Bowen, aromatherapy, Flower remedies, and other forms of healing. What makes a naturopath a true practitioner is not the modalities he/she uses, but that the modalities of healing are used to treat the fundamental cause of disease, treat the whole person, and treat each person as an individual.

There is an undefined quality to this way of practicing naturopathic medicine, which puts it in harmony with the healing power of Nature, being quite hard to define in and of itself. No one can tell a naturopath of the true art of our medicine which modalities he/she must use or in which way it is right. That decision is based on personal preference, and decided by the modalities that resonate with or excite the naturopath.

The third way of naturopathy is somewhere in between the other two. It does have the capacity to help people heal and to cure disease. This way has been around since the dawning of our medicine. It is the way of the naturopath that uses supplements, herbs, homeopathy, hydrotherapy and nutrition to get the different systems of the body working properly. It cleanses and supports the liver, gets the bowels moving, supports and tonifies the adrenals, purifies the blood. It promotes detoxification and works to get all the organs in high gear. Rather than treating the whole person, it is expert on the physical realm, treating the systems of the body, ensuring everything is properly functioning. This way of practicing naturopathy can help people feel better because it works. We will call it "systems-based naturopathy."

One advantage of whole person naturopathy over allopathic and systems-based naturopathy is its low cost. Allopathic and systems-based naturopathy are very costly, more costly than many people can afford. Naturopaths, at times, have gotten a bad name because of the immense price people pay for all the herbs and supplements they get after a visit. When you treat systems or symptoms, it becomes tempting to increase the number of supplements and herbs for more and more systems and/or symptoms. "I'll just add a little bit of this for the thyroid, a little bit of that for the bowels, some of this for the adrenals, some of these for the liver..." When you treat this way, it is easy to justify giving more and more until the person is on 10 different supplements at one time. This is an unskilled way of practicing our medicine. And it is much too expensive for many people. Some times it works, sometimes it doesn't. When it doesn't work, and people have paid hundreds of dollars and don't feel much better, they're very upset.

The whole ND, the truest practitioner of the art and science of naturopathic medicine, can incur only the cost of his/her time upon the copatient without having to charge them for all kinds of supplements and expensive tests, with modalities like homeopathy (if they have a dispensary), acupuncture (just the cost of the needles), counseling (just the cost of the air), nutrition (just the cost of the right food that people have to buy anyway), massage and other hands-on techniques like cranio-sacral, Bowen and hands-on-healing and hydrotherapy (just the cost of the water). All these modalities cost next to nothing above the practitioner's fee for his/her time. That is the beauty that naturopathic medicine and all healing modalities have that allopathic and systems-based medicine do not. The modalities themselves are almost without cost. When I think of a healing medicine that works in harmony with the healing power of Nature, I want it to be something that is relatively low in cost. Not that the practitioner asks little for his/her expertise and professional skills, because the exchange of money for service is important. Rather the idea that the healing occurs naturally, facilitated by techniques and modalities that are as seamless and costless as the healing power of Nature itself. That makes sense to me.

If the government could disentangle itself from the lobbying of the pharmaceutical industry, they would see that the solution to their health care problems, the deterioration of their hospitals and the overtaxed budget, all lies in adopting the healing paradigm and naturopathic doctors as the primary health care givers in chronic disease. All the wisdom that we possess in our profession would then be made available to the world. The cost of health care would plummet because NDs use modalities that are relatively costless. People would be happier, healthier, and wealthier.

Naturopaths would bring the health of any country up several notches by simply sharing the importance of proper exercise, the necessity of drinking adequate, clean water, and by providing healthy, natural alternatives to immunizations in children. These changes alone could reduce the incidence and cost of disease immensely. All the money spent on expensive tests in healthcare would also be greatly reduced. With people being healthier and happier and empowered within their lives, they would lead more productive lives. Every industry in the country and the country itself would benefit. Our health is intimately related to our lives. If governments would take the initiative and change their health care system from the conventional medical model to the healing model, led in part by naturopaths, the countries themselves would benefit economically and in overall well-being.

Another problem with the systems-based method is that it does work, yet it doesn't necessarily last that long, because once the supplements and herbal protocols are stopped, the person can relapse. This is also a problem of the allopathic way or any physically-based treatment, which often has a rebound effect of the symptoms becoming worse when the treatment is stopped. Because the cause of disease was not addressed, the person was not treated as a whole, and the naturopath did not act as teacher to help these people make changes in their lives that will benefit them forever. The copatient will continue to think the toxic thoughts and feel the things about themselves that caused them to get sick in the first place. Purifying the pipes is good. Supporting the body is good too. But if the person keeps the stress-response and cascade of control and resistance in their body by living the belief systems that are not harmonious with life, they are not helped in the long run by cleaning out the pipes or bolstering depleted organs. The responsibility for their own health was not put in the right place.

In a system of medicine where the doctors teach people to fish, they do not only provide a fish for a day, people do not depend on continuous health care. In addition, since they have learned to empower themselves, they will naturally rub off on the rest of the people in their environment and cause a chain reaction of people who are not needy for their health, but capable of rendering themselves well.

Another dilemma that a naturopath can face, which is not so much a problem of mixing up our philosophy but occurs because we have at our disposal so many different modalities, is the problem of "What did what?" "Was it the counseling we did together, was it the nutritional changes, or was it the homeopathic remedy?" Homeopaths scoff at this sort of approach because their medicine is so precise and so specific that it requires no other thing to improve health. The many things at once seem crude. But naturopaths do not rely on one thing only. In an initial visit, if you assess that the person is not eating well and not getting enough exercise and you suggest changes in diet and lifestyle, and they return in one month feeling much better, does it really matter what did what? Are you going to simply change the diet and wait a month to see if everything gets better because of this change? Maybe not. You might suggest the increase in exercise too. And if you had a long history and took a good homeopathic case too, perhaps you will be ready to suggest a remedy that fits their totality while you have also suggested other things.

Of course, you don't want to do too many things. And in all honesty, the singular approach is probably the wisest and most effective, especially if it zeros in on the cause, the core belief or delusion in most cases, and treats the whole person in this way. Giving one remedy or using only a few acupuncture needles can be very effective if it is not all mixed up with other forms of treatment.

However, there is another very important reason why it should not matter what did what in a case. When you take good histories and people share all levels of their being with you, they can change how they think and live because they are more aware of themselves. This has the greatest effect on their lives. Because of this ability we all have to heal ourselves, if you try to attribute the healing all to one thing, even when you give good treatments and remedies, you are taking the copatient out of the equation, much in the same way allopathic medicine does. So the need to know or believe that the treatment you suggested was the cause of the healing still involves taking the responsibility for people's health out of their own hands.

Even in homeopathy, after giving one well-selected remedy, the changes that take place can be attributed to many things. In many cases, people are sick because they are not living well, they are choosing unhealthy jobs and relationships. After taking the remedy, they leave the relationship or job and begin to feel much better. Of course the homeopath can claim it is the remedy that gave them the courage and insight to leave the situations that were harmful to them. Perhaps that is in fact what happened. But it is not for us to pinpoint exactly where the healing came from. Maybe the remedy did give a little boost or cause an immense shift, and feeling better, they began to allow themselves better things in their lives, like better exercise, food and relationships. Maybe it was just sitting in your chair talking to you, sharing their issues that gave the person the right awareness to make changes in his/her life and subsequently heal. When copatients get better, it is best to give both their ability to heal themselves and the treatment you selected the benefit of the doubt. This way, the physician remains humble before the healing power of Nature and does not play God.

Therefore, if you counsel your copatients, and you give a remedy and they are doing better and feeling better, you have done your job. As precise and understandable as it is for a homeopath or an acupuncturist to want to isolate all variables down to solely the action of the remedy or the needle, in truth, you never know for sure what did what and it doesn't really matter.

One might say that they have to know if the remedy is acting to know if they should repeat it in the future. Well, if you give a remedy and the person is doing better, even if you intervened with other modalities, like nutrition and counseling, you will try that remedy again if those symptoms are still present pointing to that same remedy.

The mixing of different modalities is possible when working within our philosophy because they all act together like the different instruments in an orchestra, bringing forward the music as a whole. You do not want to mix allopathy with whole person medicine in cases where a person is able to heal from within, or the result will be like playing two different arrangements at the same time. This causes dissonance and disharmony because the allopathic and naturopathic ways work oppositely. If you have copatients who are constipated and you counsel them to help them not to be so uptight about their jobs, their homes, or their lives in general and you find they could use Calcarea carbonica as a good remedy, don't also put them on a botanical formula of laxatives to get the bowels functioning. When our bodies stop working ideally, it is because we are not working ideally within our minds and emotions. There is stress, uptightness. Perhaps Calc-carb people get constipated so often because they are so uptight? They have an idea about life that doesn't permit them to relax. This control of the mind controls the Qi which controls the body. There is nothing wrong with the colon that is constipated. It is simply reflecting what is going on in the mind. But a constipated colon that gets commands from the mental/emotional sphere to be constipated while also receiving a laxative formula gets confused. What should I do, it asks? I am being told to be uptight and constipated by my mind and at the same time I am being forced to be loose. When someone goes on an allopathic protocol they often become worse after the protocol is stopped. The reason for this is that the body was being forced to do one thing and the command center (mind) was telling it to do exactly the opposite. The command center is obeyed most closely and persistently. During an allopathic treatment like herbal laxatives, even if the stools are helped to move, the body fights the external deliverance of herbs or supplements or whatever is treating it allopathically because it wants to be constipated. So when the laxatives are stopped, there is a rebound. It is similar to what one can observe with hypotensive drugs. A person is so stressed out that his/her blood pressure is up at around 180/120. Then the patient goes on hypotensives and the blood pressure returns to normal for a while. But it will go back to 180/120 after some time because the body means to express the high pressure in the person's stressed-out mind and after a while, the tolerance that is shown to a certain dosage of a drug demonstrates that the body has become strong *against* it. The body is just a reflection of the mind, mirroring it, copying what goes on in the mental realm. When the blood pressure returns to the original high level, even on the hypotensives, the allopathic solution to this problem is to increase the dosage. This can continue until the person is on such a high dose that he/she must then switch to another drug when the first one no longer acts.

In the Calc-carb constipation case, healing the whole person requires the cause of the constipation be treated at its root. This requires that the energy of the bowel be healed from within, at the source of the constipation in the mental/ emotional realm. Then allow the healing power of Nature to naturally bring about balance in the bowels. Even though it might seem like you are helping the person in the direction they want by giving laxatives, you are merely giving an artificial relief to the symptoms, which is fighting in the opposite direction that the body wants to go. The body will relapse as an expression of its frustration and the fact that its wishes to copy the mind were not respected or heeded.

Therefore, one can combine modalities in a whole person method, such as counseling and homeopathy or acupuncture, even if you are not sure what does what, because they work in the same direction, holistically in harmony with Nature, and help toward the ultimate goal of bringing better health to a person. But it is not useful to combine the use of allopathic treatments with holistic ones in the treatment of most chronic disease because they work in opposition.

It might be necessary to do both when someone is very sick and close to death, with little fighting vitality. In this case, it could be necessary to support the body so that you can give some strength to heal and so the patient doesn't die while you try to help him/her heal from within. Some practitioners also believe it is necessary to treat both allopathically and holistically in cancer cases. In homeopathy, this would involve finding the remedy that matches the lesion or the tumour's expression in the body, and also treating the whole person constitutionally. In other modalities, it could involve giving anti-tumour supplementation and nutrition to support the person, detoxifying the body, giving anti-oxidants, all the while addressing the root causes, the issues that have affected them for years and brought about the imbalances that led to cancer.

CHAPTER 8

The Screening Process, The Clinic and NPLEX
Aligning with the Way of Naturopathy

WHEN SOMETHING has a purpose, everything it does must be aligned and must work in harmony to help in carrying out that purpose. It is the same with our profession. All that we do, all that we use, all that we study, must be aligned with our purpose. Everything else should be transformed or released. The screening process, the clinic and NPLEX must all be aligned with the purpose of naturopathic medicine education. Whatever is in those elements or otherwise in our profession that doesn't serve us to be whole NDs must be transformed or removed. The education itself is dealt with in the next chapter.

The screening process is of utmost importance, not only because it filters out students who are not made for the profession, but also because it sets the stage in the student's mind for what is important in the entire program. As it has stood until now, the screening process has very poorly fulfilled its duty of accepting only those students who will make whole person naturopaths. It must be improved.

If students get through the screening process, they will believe themselves to be ready for their studies and for the profession. Therefore, it is crucial to grill potential students with the kinds of questions that are aligned with the philosophy of our profession to indicate what the profession is all about.

"Please tell us what the difference is between treating a disease and its symptoms and treating the whole person, the cause of disease and treating each person as an individual."

"What is the difference between the allopathic medical and the naturopathic healing model?"

If those people involved in the interview understand the difference themselves, they will be able to detect authentic replies from those that are fabricated. And of course, when a hopeful gives his/her answer, the interviewer should challenge him/her on some points to discover if the student believes what he/she is talking about or if he/she just learned what to say to specific questions in preparation for the screening interview.

"What are some of the issues facing naturopathic medicine these days?"

"Did you make any attempts to be accepted into conventional medicine?"

This second question can be helpful to screen out students who might simply go through the program thinking like medical doctors and carrying out the biomedical model in their practices. We don't want students in our program who wish to be medical doctors and have just chosen naturopathic medicine as the next best thing. The screening process should therefore investigate which students did actually apply to conventional medical schools. The fact that they did is not an absolute point against their potential entry, but does help the screeners understand whether or not this student will be able to adopt the naturopathic whole person model during their studies. If students have applied to both conventional medical schools and naturopathic schools, the odds are that the distinction in their minds as to the difference between the two medicines is not very big. That is not a good sign for their potential of getting through the naturopathic screening process.

"Have you ever been to see a naturopathic doctor or a healer? What did you go for? What was your experience like?"

"Have you begun your own healing path?"

Since there will be courses in the curriculum designed to teach students to heal themselves, this is not crucial, but will bode favourably on students who have begun their own healing processes, since they already have the most essential foundation to practice whole person naturopathy.

Answers to these and other questions in the interview could include responses such as, "I don't know," indicating that the student does not need to have an answer to everything. In fact, the entire screening process is meant to gauge the student's capacity to intuit, to connect with the heart and to think outside of the box of established science and beliefs in medicine. Thus, creative, well-rounded students are sought (even with poorer marks), and the uni-dimensional students will be screened out. None of these questions or points are meant to imply that we want students in our profession who cannot deduce logically or who are intellectually daft. It is meant to ensure that students have the dimension of the intuitive and the creative and are not just governed by their left brains in their thinking processes. Students who are governed by their left brain and are not able to enter into the vast world of the intuitive and the undefined make poorer naturopaths. They can be excellent allopathic prescribers, but not true naturopaths. It is said that those students who go through the curriculum focused on getting the best grades (and not living well-rounded lives) are often those who have difficulty working and connecting with their copatients. It is because the left brain does not help you be a healer, nor is it of any use in the improvisational dance of each unique case and interview. If people believe that cramming all sorts of information into their brains will help them heal people, they are mistaken. And that is the purpose of the screening process; to limit the number of students who do not have the making of a healer before they waste their time, the college's time, and their copatients' time when they get into the clinic.

Limiting students who cannot step out of their rational minds will also limit the number of allopathic naturopaths in our profession. Those very rational students usually will not go on their own healing processes and so they will have little idea of how to help a person heal themselves and how to guide them through letting go of the cause of their illness. The only alternative for them is allopathic naturopathy, which is part of the profession, but is not a large portion of our profession's foundation and make-up.

No screening process is ever perfect and students will always squeeze through who are not really meant to be naturopaths, but if the intention behind the process is to filter out students who do not wish to learn the way of healing and the undefined principles in our philosophy, then at least it will set the stage for students to understand what is required of them and what the profession is all about during the curriculum. It will also minimize the problem of students claiming that they don't have to heal themselves or understand the healing process because it is not in the curriculum. The screening process will show them that the healing process is part of the profession, and the principles of our philosophy are important. The curriculum and examination system, of course, must then do the same.

NPLEX is another big factor that is not aligned with our profession's philosophy and either must be transformed, or removed completely. Firstly, the whole examination system of NPLEX is an exact reproduction of the allopathic way of medicine. Except for the practical exams testing skills in physical examination and in each modality of naturopathic treatment, the NPLEX is filled with allopathic questions. Even the questions on the modalities like nutrition and botanical medicine are posed in an allopathic manner. How do you treat colitis? What is a good treatment protocol for migraines, ADD, constipation? Nowhere on the NPLEX are students tested to see their rapport with their copatients, to put their good listening skills and case-taking to the test, to demonstrate their understanding of naturopathic principles, to display their creative expression as a naturopathic doctor. There is especially no test of a clinician's ability to treat the whole person, to treat each person as an individual. In all truth, it is not easy to have a written exam to do that. For that reason, NPLEX doesn't serve to align naturopathic medicine with its essence.

It is not wise to consider naturopathic students ready to practice simply for the fact that they can memorize and answer multiple-choice questions. The information that is tested on NPLEX is often not useful in practice, and even if it is, it can be accessed through reference materials and textbooks and need not be tested through memorization.

As much as our curriculum taxes students with overabundant left-brain courses, NPLEX drives the nail into the coffin. Second-year NPLEX cuts up the much-needed break between second and third-year. Fourth-year NPLEX comes after the clinic year, when students have just graduated from the program, and then requires graduates to cram 15 subjects into their brain to answer multiple choice questions. The fact that these exams are comprised of multiple-choice questions should be enough to indicate the absurdity of using such an examination system to ensure that our doctors are prepared for practice. Perhaps they are prepared to practice like medical doctors, whose method of treatment revolves around formula-based treatments for specific diseases. Have not the students demonstrated their capacity to memorize for exams by having procured university degrees? All students demonstrate by passing the NPLEX exams is their capacity to memorize information. This doesn't indicate that they are ready for practice. Our profession must dispel the illusion that such exams serve toward proving a naturopath's legitimacy. The truth about NPLEX is that they are just a way to make our profession feel better in the face of our insecurities at being a non-established profession. Saying that we are a licensed profession, that we have licensing exams, gives us a sense of security. Do we ever tell people what those exams are comprised of? NPLEX as it is now doesn't serve toward bringing out naturopathic medicine as it is conceived to be.

Our naturopaths must have faith in themselves enough to know that it doesn't matter if they have not memorized the symptoms of certain diseases or what supplements or herbs treat what condition. It is shocking for someone to think that a medical doctor doesn't know everything off by heart because our society still believes medical doctors are responsible for our health. Being responsible, medical doctors are taught to know it all and are tested to ensure that they do. Naturopaths are not responsible for people's health and so they are also not responsible to know the details about the definitions of disease and the specifics of other things like the actions of remedies, herbs or supplements. Through practice, these things become second nature. And since we go through the courses of what we need to know, then we are wise enough to know that we can consult the books we used in our studies *anytime* we need to know an answer. We can open and research books before, during, and after our consultations. Most of us are not in emergency situations, so we don't need to have memorized all the information we will ever need. Shed the need to appear as if you know it all, and you will relieve yourself of a lot of unnecessary pressure, including the unnecessary burden of memorizing for exams that emulates another system of thinking.

It is a very simple thing to say that you don't know an answer and that you must look it up. Trust that you are a good healer and you won't need to know everything or to put on the air as if you do (because there is no such thing as knowing everything anyway). If you are afraid to portray yourself as not knowing everything, you are likely buying into the model of thinking that says a doctor must know it all. Must we continue to use this method of licensing our students that is clearly not aligned with our profession's essence?

Our profession's choice to be recognized and legitimized within a model of medicine that is not our own has created a curriculum that is very stressful for students, who sometimes become sick from it. Our students begin the four-year program excited, hopeful, and full of energy and sometimes leave feeling burnt out. Some students get sick during the program and it takes years to recover. The NPLEX only makes these matters worse. Prolonged left-brained study is not healthy. Pouring over books and memorizing facts causes one's energy to be focused up in the brain in the very same way that fear and stress do. Even if students are not stressed out by the prospect of having repeated exams for several days in a row, they will feel stress as they lose the connection with their bodies by spending so much time focusing with their brain. The goal of most healing meditations and spiritual practice is to stop the process of being overly rational, of always thinking, and being so cerebral. But studying for exams like NPLEX makes such matters worse and leads to disharmony. The program, teaching students to heal, to help improve people's health by releasing the harmful stress of their lives, should not stress students out.

The NPLEX also looms over the four-year program menacingly because students are taught, "You need this for NPLEX," and they study it because they need to know it to pass an exam and be granted a license, not because of how the information will help them work with the healing power of Nature. The courses are often designed specifically to prepare students for this allopathic exam. This definitely contributes to the mutation of our curriculum into something that serves the fear we have of being illegitimate, rather than of being ourselves.

I would prefer people come to see me because I am a good naturopath rather than making their decision to see me based on the fact that I have a license. If our copatients only knew how little our license speaks to our capacity as true naturopathic doctors!

Thus NPLEX must change to incorporate the examination of subtle skills like listening, non-judgmentalness, and whole person assessment and guidance. Live cases should be part of the exams that demonstrate students' readiness to graduate. NPLEX could continue to test the physical skills we have learned like acupuncture needling, manipulation, and other hands on skills. But if you really think about it, there is no reason that the colleges could not conduct these exams before students graduate. The colleges could take the responsibility of testing all naturopathic skills and be ultimately responsible for graduation of their students. Therefore, NPLEX really is not serving any extraordinary service toward creating well-balanced, whole person naturopaths. It simply emulates another way of thinking. It stresses students out by testing them in ways that indicate very little.

Our profession is self-regulated. The things that we have chosen to do to legitimize ourselves are by our own hands, our own choices. Nobody forces us to create a curriculum and an examination system that is allopathic so that we will seem credible. It is our choice. Being so, we can design the process of licensing to be perfectly aligned with our philosophy to ensure that those graduating are ready to practice whole person naturopathic medicine, and are capable of referencing materials properly when required. Thus, nobody is going to mind (but ourselves) if we purge ourselves of NPLEX in order to realign our program and profession with our principles.

For all those graduates in positions of authority in the colleges, as board members and on councils, please do not say, "I suffered, so should you!" to keep NPLEX. Sometimes people who are raised in a tough environment feel the need to create toughness for those who follow them even if the toughness is pointless. This feeling will also exist in our profession amongst the graduates that suffered and succeeded in passing all their NPLEX. There is a sense of accomplishment that is rightly felt. But those who have succeeded in passing NPLEX must now also understand the importance of dissolving NPLEX.

To some, without NPLEX, the program might seem too easy and lacking the challenge necessary for students' growth. This I see as a sort of, "No pain. No gain," philosophy that is dated and doesn't work toward raising naturopaths who can feel the subtle workings of the healing power of Nature. And the four-year program will still be packed with many demanding courses and the incredible challenge of self-healing. Growing into a healer, a whole ND, will never be easy. But the proper growth of a naturopath in an environment that is in harmony with his/her true nature will bring joy and a sense of purpose and enthusiasm. It will not deplete but invigorate. Ridding ourselves of NPLEX is a decision that will best serve the profession.

The clinic is at the forefront of representing both the profession and the education. It is the looking glass for naturopathic medicine and the arena for students to train and practice naturopathy. It is the threshold of the education that will have a great effect on the student's future in our medicine. As such, it must be closely maintained in alignment with the true philosophy and essence of our medicine.

In the clinic, we set the stage for what is the acceptable professional behaviour by being who we are. Since that is quite broad in scope, the professional behaviour and façade witnessed in the clinic and the rest of the college should be a reflection of Nature's myriad ways of expressing Herself. If we emulate the professionalism of other professions, then our demeanor is forced and overly proper, like our political correctness can be. It looks phony and can leave people visiting the clinic wondering what naturopathic medicine really is. The confusion of identity of our profession becomes evident in our clinic. Even if people cannot put their fingers on what was wrong while they visited the clinic, they leave with an empty feeling, like they just went to a dinner with recent graduates of a school of correction.

When people are true to themselves, no matter how strange they might seem compared to an established norm, that authenticity has a strong, clear quality. It is also wonderful to witness and is irresistible. It inspires others to let down their masks and their falsified behaviour. The whole world suffers from a fear of being itself. We owe it to humanity to demonstrate the joy and freedom that comes from creative self-expression. This is the calling of the naturopath; to be true on all fronts, on all levels. This is the healing we need in our program and our clinics. I long to see naturopathic students allowed to be free to express themselves as they see fit in the corridors of the school, and the halls, and rooms of the clinic.

I remember I was skipping down the halls of our clinic, singing, looking anything but "professional." I don't think I even had my lab coat on at the time, and somehow I had forgotten to put on my necktie. One of the other clinicians was pushing an older lady-copatient in a wheelchair. They both saw me skip past them like a king's jester. Later that day, the other clinician told me that the old lady had said, "I love you naturopathic doctors" in response to my "unprofessional" behaviour.

The environment where any form of healing takes place should be free and joyous for all people to express themselves as they are, not conforming to a demeanor that has a certain definition of proper and professional.

It is also essential that the supervisors in the clinics be naturopathic doctors who have the understanding of our philosophy, who have been through the process of self-healing and who understand the undefined dance of individual, whole person and underlying-cause medicine. Having been through the process of healing, they will understand the issues that arise in the clinician when he/she begins to work with the first copatients: the insecurities, the saviour-complexes, the fear of doing the wrong thing, saying the wrong thing, prescribing the wrong thing. The supervisors are not just there to verify treatment protocols and ensure safety, but to support and encourage students to trust themselves, to trust what they know and their skills as healers. The clinic is a growing process, a process of being encouraged in the baby steps of naturopathic practice, not a process where everyone needs to conform to what the supervisors say and suggest. Not all supervisors, even the allopathic ones, will dictate the protocols that students carry out. But some supervisors make the error of letting students rely too heavily on their knowledge. It is a natural thing to want to lean on somebody who knows more than you. This method of learning impedes the necessary growth of trust and confidence that clinicians must have in order to embrace their own expressions of healing and naturopathy—as stated on page 43 of the HOA, "a knowledge of their unique skills as healers…" If students do not come to understand their unique skills as healers during time in the clinic, when they get out in their own practice, they will end up leaning on that which is laid out for them, proven, and clearly delineated.

When naturopaths begin practicing, it is natural to experience fears and insecurities. If naturopathic clinicians are not supported and encouraged to find their own paths and to align with naturopathic philosophy, they will lean on formula-based medicine. It is the formulas of "give this herb or supplement for that condition." In the insecurity of beginning clinic, without the proper guidance and encouragement of the supervisors, the clinician will adopt the allopathic paradigm of medicine and treat the symptoms of disease or the disease itself, because that way is already established and "proven." This is easy and provides fewer risks. The supervisors must be strict in not allowing this where it is not necessary. They must ensure that a student is treating the individual, finding what is unique about the copatient on all levels, helping empower that copatient to make different choices, change beliefs, and act in harmony with the spontaneous healing power of Nature. Such growth of a student in this way, over the course of the year, gives a sense of self and confidence in his/her own healing abilities. When one leans on the crutch of allopathic treatment, one has no confidence in his/her own abilities as a whole ND. This can threaten and frighten a naturopathic out on his/her own. Thus the responsibility falls on the clinic to certify the proper growth of students into whole NDs while they are still growing in the clinic.

Since the clinic is a reflection of the curriculum, allopathic naturopathy makes up the majority of treatment seen in the clinic. This carries over from all the allopathic teaching. Or, perhaps it is the lack of holistic training during the curriculum that makes students default into allopathy in the clinic. What choice do they have? Therefore, to see the students practicing the essence of their medicine, it will require that the essence become reestablished in the curriculum.

Aligning the screening process, NPLEX and the clinic with our roots and the principles of our philosophy plays a necessary part toward growing efficient, skilled naturopathic doctors. The most essential place to do so lies in the education of the curriculum.

CHAPTER 9

The Education

Part I: The Standards of Naturopathic Education

The Council of Naturopathic Medical Education (CNME), the accreditation agency for naturopathic medicine, began in 1978, when the two existing colleges at that time, NCNM and Bastyr, were defenders and protectors of the faith of naturopathic philosophy and principles. The CNME had no need to establish definitive standards that described the essence of naturopathic medicine and how a school needed to conform its program in line with the unique attributes of naturopathic medicine because that was the very basis of the program. The CNME concentrated instead on making sure the schools were respectable institutions of higher education and that they ran themselves professionally.

As time passed, there was more interest in starting naturopathic schools from people outside the profession. Some of the existing schools had key administrators who were not NDs themselves. The CNME is aware now that they can no longer take for granted that a naturopathic college is a true subscriber to the basic tenets of naturopathic medicine. In addition, the CNME favours naturopathic medicine embracing its path. Currently, there are thirteen seats on the Council. Seven of these seats are naturopathic doctors, most of whom were raised in the profession when the education focused entirely around the philosophy of our medicine. They are now interested in seeing the profession aligned with its roots.

We are at an interesting time. Never before has our profession been so close to recognition by the governments of Canada and the U.S.. Never before have the colleges been so professional and so consistent with the standards of higher education. What is essential now is to fill the structure/shell that the colleges have become with the guts that make up our profession. And so should the voices of naturopathic students be expressed to the colleges and the CNME. The CNME has an excellent policy of recognizing and reviewing all complaints and concerns written both by students in the core of the program and naturopaths in the field. The power in numbers of people corroborating to see all aspects of the program acting in harmony with our philosophy will help CNME ensure that the colleges keep with the program. So we all have a voice in the formation of our medicine. Soon we will see students being excited and invigorated by the program as they grow into the NDs they long to be.

Until then, there are a few points about our education and curriculum to examine that would help us align with the essence of the profession.

As long as the main criteria for competency in the program are being met, the CNME allows the colleges some leeway in the development of the curriculum, encouraging uniqueness in the different colleges. Some core curriculum decisions are being made at the level of colleges that influence the standard of naturopathic education and are not in accordance with the ideal for naturopathic education. For example, most of the colleges are making errors now in accepting too many students per year. Having a higher student intake provides a financial boost to the colleges. Students are seen as dollar signs. It is a natural instinct of any institution to want to thrive financially. But this must be kept in balance or the integrity of the education gets compromised.

The number of students in a classroom for learning the healing paradigm, for sharing in a safe, open setting, for counseling, acupuncture, homeopathy, etc., should not exceed 40. Having 50 in one class is stretching it, but can be manageable. If the classes are too big, the subtleties of the art of our medicine cannot be properly applied. Right brain learning requires many questions to be answered by an experienced, knowledgeable instructor/practitioner. The questions do not have a black and white answer because the medicine is not black and white. Naturopathic education must be provided in a way that instructs students to be able to understand the essence of the medicine, allowing them to learn the core of the undefined, fluid form of healing that they can then apply in their unique ways. Having too many students does not encourage this kind of learning. Having too many students encourages the black and white, rational learning of bits and pieces of information and mimicking established thinking. Therefore, if 150 students are admitted every year, they must be split entirely into A, B and C classes, depending on the overall number of students per year. This requires more teachers, more staff and more resources. That is most likely not possible or reasonable, which might also be a good thing, because having 150 students per year brings up another dilemma, which is related to the screening process. If the number of accepted students is between 120 and 150 and the number of total applicants is around 200 (which is the approximate yearly average for the colleges), the ratio is quite low; between 10:1 and 1N:1. Many of these students accepted into the colleges are not really made to be naturopathic doctors. Some were the non-accepted students from conventional medicine; others are just looking for a profession. These students do not make good Nature doctors.

The profession is still in its baby steps. Things that grow too quickly and do not have a proper foundation always crumble. This is the danger of graduating so many insufficiently prepared naturopathic doctors who do not understand the essence of the medicine. The profession must grow slowly, from the roots, with a smaller number of graduates who represent the medicine in its pure form. When the success of the profession grows and the awareness of the public increases such that there are many more students applying every year and the profession is thriving financially, then we can afford to have a larger number of students. Until then, the overall intake of the college should be reduced to about 40–50 students per year. This number increases the ratio of applicants to accepted students and is a better number for the quality of the education. This way, the colleges will graduate 40 or 50 good doctors, rather than 150 weaker ones.

There is a solution to this issue that provides both the financial stability and growth of the institution while maintaining the integrity and essence of naturopathic education. Dr. Chris Sowton, N.D., suggested it to me. It is the jewel of the crown concept and the idea is as follows: The college provides many different peripheral programs ranging from certificate programs to singular courses to educate the public in the various fields of knowledge that naturopathic medicine offers: Homeopathy, acupuncture and Tradition Chinese Medicine, botanical medicine, nutrition, hydrotherapy, nutritional supplementation, cranio-sacral therapy, midwifery, etc. The school can even provide programs for Yoga, Pilates, and meditation. The income from these peripheral programs (the crown), enables the college to have a jewel program of 40–50 students who go through the core ND degree. The pressure of the institution to survive financially is alleviated by the income from the peripheral programs. The overall cost of the jewel program can also be decreased so that it doesn't become prohibitive to the students who cannot afford the ever-increasing costs.

The core, jewel program will entice the students participating in the fringe programs to become interested in the jewel: the naturopathic medicine program. The people interested in the peripheral program will also be more mature students, self-motivated and with more life experience (since they voluntarily will be seeking additional knowledge and will likely have already graduated from university). They will be better equipped to become naturopathic doctors capable of working independently, thinking for themselves, and recognizing the importance of self-development and self-healing in order to embrace the subtleties of the medicine. Dr. Sowton's jewel of the crown idea provides solutions to the problems of accepting too many students into the core of the program and the financial concerns that the colleges have by accepting fewer students.

Another problem of our education is that the standards we set for ourselves are standards of education that do not necessary work in harmony with naturopathic learning. Seeking accreditation is a noble cause, but not when it compromises the essence of a profession. We seek high standards in our education, yet those standards are being adopted from other professions. Naturopathic medicine is unique and must not emulate standards of other education systems, but establish its own standards. It is a better idea to set the standards of naturopathic education according to what will create the best NDs, fluid Nature doctors capable of working in harmony with the Vis and healing the whole person. Recognition from the public and government will follow. This is something we must trust, instead of seeking recognition by emulating a standard that ultimately compromises the integrity of our medicine.

The CNME is seeking recognition by the U.S. Secretary of Education. All the criteria that the CNME seeks to fulfill are criteria that the U.S. Secretary of Education recognizes as high standards in education. Those high standards have been established in the rationally-based education systems of the past. There is no precedent for intuitive learning, for students learning to heal themselves, or for the kind of environment that is optimal for teaching our modalities. When teaching the essence of homeopathy or acupuncture, for instance, what standard does the government of the U.S. possess with which to compare? When studying homeopathy, questions about the specifics of prescription, selecting remedies, and dosing, are often met with the answer "It depends," because each case is different, each situation special. Our medicine is equally special and our education must reflect that. Seeking accreditation in another's standards is like dressing up in a stiff costume. Can you walk truly and freely?

One of Naturopathic medicine's purposes is to help change the way people think about medicine. The philosophy of our medicine is distinctive from currently established medicine and our education should reflect that. Comparing our medicine to the way of thinking of a standard University or establishment of Higher Education will not work either, because the universities are built upon a foundation of rational thought, and naturopathic medicine works best and in harmony with Nature, with a right-brained education acting as its foundation. The fact alone that over 70% of naturopathic students are women should tell us that our education's content should not be rationally dominant and geared toward men, who were the ones to create the education and who were, historically, the only ones allowed to study.

As we now begin to focus on suffusing the heart of naturopathy into the standards for higher education, the curriculum must have teachers who are experienced in practice and who trust the healing process and understand it enough to convey it to the students. In the colleges, the standards of higher education are being met with well-educated teachers, yet, not being naturopaths, they have no sense of whole person healing. This perpetuates the allopathic and left-brain model of medicine on students. The other situation is due to the fact that many recent graduates get teaching positions. Coming from a largely allopathic program, they understand the allopathic paradigm more than anything else and convey this to the students. These students are graduating and doing the same so the situation snowballs. The colleges must pay experienced naturopaths enough to entice them to teach. This is one of the most essential points that the CNME should ensure for the standard of our education—good, experienced, whole ND teachers. A good teacher can turn a dull subject into an inspiring one. A good naturopath who understands the healing power of Nature, in addition to being able to teach the essence of naturopathic medicine, can also suffuse the science courses with naturopathic content to make the subjects interesting and relevant to practice.

Another way in which we must not adapt to the way of the world is in the definition of what it means to be primary health care physicians. I feel that naturopathic doctors must absolutely be primary health care physicians or we will not have a future. However, we must redefine primary health care around our medicine and not adapt to conventional medicine's definition of it.

Looking at naturopathic primary health care is very simple. It involves treating *people* with all manifestations of disease—from migraines and depression, to hepatitis and cancer. Our future is assured when we do so in a manner that is holistic and in harmony with our philosophy. As we discussed the elements of conventional medicine from which we must detach in the previous chapters, our redefined primary health care need not involve diagnosing or treating disease, nor does it involve the prognosis of disease. Naturopathic doctors are responsible for being caring, kind, and aware in practice, but are not responsible for copatients' health. If we are truly responsible for only one thing, it is to teach people that they are responsible for their own health and that their health is in their own hands. This is not a cop-out, nor is it shying away from the challenge of primary health care. Rather it is taking up the challenge of creating a new territory where the healing power of Nature works best, unopposed by misconceptions about healing and medicine that keep people bound to their illness.

So to state clearly the question, "As primary health care physicians, should naturopathic doctors have to differentially diagnose disease?" I believe that the answer to this question is "No." Often people seek naturopathic care after a diagnosis from conventional medicine. The exceptional cases that need to be treated allopathically that do not have a differential diagnosis can be referred to conventional medicine for diagnosis. That is how naturopathic medicine and conventional medicine can work beautifully together. Primary health care need not represent absolute autonomy over health, where a naturopath has to play the role of medical doctor and healer. Even family doctors, who have always been regarded as primary health care practitioners, are constantly referring their patients for diagnostic tests.

If naturopathic medicine concerns itself too much with preparing students to be capable of differentially diagnosing, and the accreditation process sets that as its standard, it will have to emulate the rest of conventional medical study as well. This is dabbling too much outside of the essence of our medicine, which, as a reminder, is to treat the root, the individual, and the whole person, not the disease. The diagnosis of disease is not a subject in which you can dabble. Either you focus greatly on it and become as competent as medical doctors, or you recognize the fact that naturopathic primary health care does not require disease diagnosis. If we continue to attempt to be competent enough for diagnosis of disease, we will be competing with conventional medicine, where we do not stand a chance. We shouldn't compete in diagnosis because it is not our realm and will compromise the essence of our medicine by spending too much time in the allopathic model.

The only alternative is to have a six-year program, so that students can become expert at differential diagnosis and also have enough time to learn and become what naturopathic medicine is about. I don't see this as a good direction for naturopathic medicine to take. We will not be tapping properly into the pure form of our medicine in this way. When someone recognizes the healing power of Nature, understands its subtleties, and trusts in its processes, they no longer focus on disease and its treatment. That is the goal we must set for our profession as well. The confusion in naturopathic medicine creates confusion between allopathic and naturopathic paradigms in the curriculum. If we emphasis allopathic diagnosis and treatment with the healing power of Nature, we still have not recognized the Vis and we will create a distortion in our profession.

Medicine is not something to practice in fear. The association of primary health, in naturopathic medicine, with the need to diagnose disease is rooted in the fear of missing a diagnosis. This fear influences the definition of primary health to such an extent that our entire curriculum and accreditation process become affected by it. This fear comes from the belief that doctors are responsible for their patients' health. The fear is also associated with believing that, "Doing no harm," means not missing the manifestations of disease that can acutely or dangerously affect a person. Naturopathic doctors and healers are not responsible for people's health. Does that sound irresponsible? It is not. When people start learning on a broad scale that they should not expect a doctor to take care of them, but rather that they should go to a doctor to help them heal themselves, the health of the entire planet will improve. The exorbitant cost of health care will decline, people will not fear disease but will learn from it, and they will not hold their doctors liable for their health conditions.

For this reason, naturopathic education should not concern itself so much with courses that are geared toward diagnosing and treating disease. The CNME must assure that naturopaths are not just taking the reins of conventional medicine and riding the same horse, practicing green allopathic medicine.

Certain conditions still wave a red flag when someone exhibits signs of them. Acute appendicitis, threatening myocardial infarct, angina that does not ameliorate with rest, neurological disturbances such as loss of vision or speech and loss of sensation in certain parts of the body, fainting spells, are some examples of red flag conditions that should be dealt with immediately. Dealing with acute conditions that can result in death or serious complications remains within conventional medicine's scope of practice. Naturopaths must know when to recognize these conditions and know when to refer. It does not require the entire curriculum to prepare a student to recognize the red flags, nor must a student be able to diagnose all disease. It takes only one specialized course teaching students when to recognize the conditions that are serious enough to threaten a copatient's life—perhaps called the "Red Flag" course. Graduating NDs will remain primary health care physicians and *be safe practitioners*. The rest of the education can then focus on building students up to know that they have all the tools they need in their whole person naturopathy toolbox to deal with most people's manifestation of disease.

It is not just doctors who should be educated in recognizing red flag conditions, but the general public should learn when to recognize the signs and symptoms of diseases that can rapidly aggravate or deteriorate. Then people will again have the ability to spot these conditions in themselves and others and can rely less on their doctor.

Patterns of belief systems do not change overnight. Copatients might keep coming back with the notion that you, the ND, are responsible for their health, especially if naturopathic medicine does not make it clear to the public that we place responsibility for health in the hands of the patient. As the number of NDs who truly understand their role in treating individuals in the root of their illness and on all levels of their being grows, it will not take long for the public to understand this new way of thinking.

When you pour Nature's healing power into an area, all that needs to heal will transform and take on a better balance and relationship with Nature. The same is true for our education. How can we expect to carry out our purpose and develop our students properly if our education is not in harmony with its roots? Let us look at this incongruity between our essence and our education. When the foundation of our education encourages the growth of whole NDs, we will be ready to help people adapt to a new way. This way, when the CNME writes a proposal for recognition by the U.S. Secretary of Education, it will explain the uniqueness of our medicine in a way that helps the government understand that it is a safe and necessary way of educating naturopathic students.

Soon our governments will recognize naturopathy as a legitimate medicine. It is best that they recognize us when we are being true to ourselves and not because we conformed to gain credibility. The public voice will also continue to rise, encouraging the governments to recognize alternative forms of medicine as legitimate and safe.

Part II: Making Room in the Curriculum for What Counts

It would be nice to be able to accommodate every single subject in the biomedical world and have all the naturopathic courses crammed into the curriculum. But this just doesn't work. Naturopathic students are already overworked and don't have enough time to develop the proper skills in our naturopathic modality courses and the essence of the medicine. Medical students take 18–23 credits per quarter. Naturopathic students take 28 credits per quarter. One of the solutions to this problem involves making the core education program one year longer. This is not the best solution. It is the desire to make the curriculum larger to accommodate all the excess courses that are not in harmony with our medicine, and that are still attached to another model of both education and medicine. Having the curriculum one year longer still keeps the education divided between allopathic and naturopathic and graduates students who are confused between the two models of medicine.

The core naturopathic education would be better off instead by focusing completely on developing NDs capable of working whole person medicine in harmony with our philosophy. All allopathic protocols and methods will then be offered as exceptional classes, giving the correct impression that this is a rare application of the medicine. The courses that are offered should at least have merit in the clinical setting. All the space taken up by courses that do not serve whole naturopathy must be dismissed to make room for more important courses; courses that bring students substance and help them grow into healers.

The jewel program of naturopathic medicine, being comprised of mature students interested in personal growth, self-healing, and capable of self-motivating, will enable much room to be made in the curriculum, with many courses released or the number of hours decreased, because the students are capable of referencing materials and researching the information that they require.

If one is interested in the information of courses that are no longer part of the core education program, there are ample sources. We are in the age of information. There are books and courses available at various educational institutions to supplement one's knowledge. With the advantage of simply surfing or accessing databases on the Internet, we have information at our fingertips. It is no longer necessary to sit through entire courses that go through the details of left-brain information that is easily forgotten. Students can be brought through the various subjects, learning what information is contained in which courses, and how to reference that material if the need arises. All courses must also be presented in ways that challenge the student to think clinically and as whole NDs.

If some courses are still deemed necessary for students to brush up on at least once, they can also be made a pre-requisite. If students have already done the course once, as part of their undergraduate degree or as a prerequisite, then the course does not need to be repeated in the curriculum. Learning a course once is sufficient. We need not learn and forget the same things three times over, like the Krebs cycle, which I learned in Cegep, then forgot, then relearned in University, then forgot, then learned again at naturopathic college, and now have forgotten again. But I can always look it up and remind myself of its pleasurable intricacies, if I ever feel the need.

We must remember to let go of things that don't serve. It is not that we don't like the knowledge that these courses can impart. Any knowledge is nice. But just as when you clean up the garage to make room, you have to let go of the junk that only takes up space. That old bike that you haven't ridden for 20 years, but is oh so nostalgic, has got to go. The baby pool you used to splash in. It might hurt for a bit, but once you let them go, you become aware of the necessity of doing so, and you see it was a good decision.

Some of these courses that we clear from the curriculum we don't even have to replace with new ones. We can just make room… to breathe, to heal, to have less time sitting in a classroom. Some students enter the college feeling like healers and leave feeling like they couldn't help a scratch on someone's arm. And that isn't because they had to wipe the slate clean to learn the ways of healing. It is because their true essence, their core, was buried beneath all the medical model courses.

The following courses are ones that we can let go of to make room for what is truly needed in our profession. They can either be completely removed, revised in some way to take less time, or transformed to be aligned with our roots.

Histology: It is interesting to see the makeup of the various cells, but one doesn't use this information in practice. It takes up time and energy that can be devoted elsewhere. If students or naturopaths wish to use technology like dark-field microscopy in their practices, or do research involving the understanding of the histology of the cell, they can take the course themselves. This course is not useful for our curriculum and can be dismissed.

Immunology: It is nice to know how the T cells interact with the B cells and how the natural killer (NK) cells work in our bodies. However, the way the course is being taught now is not aligned with the healing paradigm. Knowing the minute details of such things is a mechanistic way of pulling the body apart into tiny components. This doesn't serve a person in treating the individual, or the cause of disease. If the details of the course are presented at all, they could be presented in a way whereby students are taught how to reference details such as what the receptors of the various cells of the immune system respond to. To align the curriculum with its roots, this course could be taught in a way that shows students what strengthens and weakens the immune system. This class could go into discussion about what diseases are related to the immune system, such as autoimmune, cancer, and HIV/AIDS. This is a course where the mind-body connection can be closely examined by looking at how the mental/emotional state affects the functioning of the immune system. Even many lay people recognize the fact that they get sick when they are stressed or feeling depressed. This course also conjures up a way in which naturopathic medicine can use science to further explain the mind-body connection, and how the immune system is affected by our thoughts and feelings.

Biochemistry: The way this course is currently presented makes naturopathic students ask, "What am I doing in this program again?" Knowing the Krebs cycle and how many ATPs are produced in oxidative phosphorylation is not useful in clinic. This course can serve a naturopathic function by looking at the biochemistry of a detox reaction, or the biochemistry of a healing crisis. The biochemistry of nutrition and digestion would also be perfect for this course, as would looking at the biochemistry of fasting, in order to educate students in the most efficient and safest way to fast. Optimal dosing of vitamins, the biochemistry of vitamin absorption and usage, and the picture of vitamin deficiencies could be perfect for this course. Orthomolecular medicine and the treatment of certain conditions with high doses of vitamins might fit nicely in this course as well.

Microbiology: All of the conditions and diseases caused by bacterial, viral and fungal microbes could be dealt with in Pathology. When this course examines the details of different microbes, it is not relevant to practice. When the bugs are covered in Pathology, students can be taught to properly reference this material when the need arises. Gonorrhea—"What microbes cause that?" Look up the bugs associated with the disease if you feel it is significant. This is another course that can be completely dismissed.

Ethics & Jurisprudence: This course is so boring that students rarely attend. Make a package of the necessary information that students need to know and can read, and then get rid of the course. Besides, teaching students about ethics will not determine if they are ethical or not. You don't want NDs behaving in a certain manner because it is unethical to behave in another. You want NDs' behaviour with copatients to come from their hearts. A curriculum that promotes and nourishes self-healing and a program that teaches students to love and accept themselves, creates naturopathic doctors that behave ethically in a natural fashion because they have learned the most valuable lessons in the world—how to care and to love. A heartfelt person is the safest and most ethical person to be around. Let the ethics and jurisprudence take the guise of classes and exercises that teach students to be good people because they are and to love themselves and all people, and to awaken their sensitivity to their copatients. This is another course to remove from the curriculum.

Pharmacology: The number of hours of this course could be reduced by not going into the detail of all the drugs and their mode of action. Studying the drugs (associated conditions, adverse effects) that people are most often on would be more relevant for practice. For any other drug, a thorough understanding of how to use the CPS could be included, along with training of how to research the information necessary for the specific drugs that are seen in a given case.

We are not learning how to use the drugs as if we want to prescribe them, but how to deal with the withdrawal, overdose symptoms, and the other effects (emotional/psychological) that occur due to the use of drugs. This course could also deal with helping copatients come off their drugs. Drugs control symptoms, but even more than that, they control the people taking them. Often when people are on drug treatment, it straightjackets them to their disease, causing a dependency on the drug to make them feel better and sometimes, to believe they need the drug to survive. Often, the person can be on a drug thinking they need to be on it for the rest of their lives. Most whole person healing only works optimally once people come off their drugs. Often the drug is just keeping all the symptoms in check, which is a kind of suppression that perpetuates disease even while controlling its symptoms. As people age, and more and more systems begin to slow and malfunction, people are put on more and more drugs. It becomes a nightmare to try to treat someone holistically when they are on so many meds. They often feel sick from all the meds, not from their original conditions. Sometimes stopping all the drugs helps the copatient feel dramatically better. In some cases, the obstacle to cure is due to the meds people are on, which they no longer need, especially if they have to come to see you for holistic medicine.

This course can help the naturopathic student understand how to help copatients come off their drugs, how to communicate with MDs to facilitate their understanding of the alternative and how to counsel people to trust the switch from the allopathic to the holistic healing paradigm. It is very rare that a copatient needs to remain on a drug, especially in cases of anxiety, depression, and other mental/emotional conditions, as well as in many other conditions, like high blood pressure, stomach acid reflux, and constipation, when the person's vitality enables the Vis to work through them. I wouldn't recommend that patients come off their drugs on their own, unless they do it gradually, are aware of their capability to heal themselves, and have the wish to be drug-free. But the goal of the naturopath should be to facilitate as many of their copatients coming off their meds as possible.

This course must also deal with harmful drug interactions with certain botanicals and supplements. This information is important when a naturopath works with physical supplements and vitamins that do have potentially harmful side effects. This is not a concern with our more energetic treatment modalities like homeopathy, acupuncture, Bach and other flower remedies, counseling, hydrotherapy, cranio-sacral, massage, all of which pose no threat of harmful inter-actions. They also do not pose the threat of poisoning patients or causing toxic side effects because of their subtle energetic nature. They are "Do no harm" friendly.

Chiropractic: The overwhelming statistics have told us what to do about this course. Around 2% of all graduates perform chiroprac-tic in their practices. It is a hands-on skill that professional chiro-practors learn exclusively for four years and that naturopathic students only dabble in. The other professions who specialize in a certain one of our modalities also do so exclusively for many more hours than we deal with them. But chiropractic is a hands-on tech-nique, where one performs the action in a succinct manner and does not have the opportunity to consult a book or a colleague. It is a tool to know how to adjust someone's neck and back, but it is not used much anymore amongst naturopathic physicians. This suggests that we do not trust our minimal training enough to use this technique to heal our patients. Perhaps we have enough other modalities that we do not need this one. Perhaps it says also that many of the stu-dents and grads do not like this technique because it can be aggres-sive and it forces against the state of the body.

Perhaps it is for these reasons that our profession is not embrac-ing chiropractic any longer. In the naturopathic profession, chiro-practic might just be a relic of the history of our profession that we are reluctant to throw away. We were closely associated with the chi-ropractors. Like the red tricycle that we loved so much still sitting in our garage, we have to say goodbye to chiropractic. It doesn't make sense for us to spend any more time studying it. Either we do it full fledge, or not at all. We cannot afford to spend any more time on it or we might as well call our program a chiropractic program. Those who wish to use chiropractic in their practice can do the advanced standing chiropractic program at a chiropractic college, just as so many chiropractors have done through the years at naturopathic col-leges. This is another course that can be completely dismissed.

Radiology (Diagnostic Imaging): Radiology goes out the door with chiropractic. The study of X-rays is also not a skill that you pick up after a few hours pouring over X-rays. You either devote a lot of time to becoming an expert, or you don't waste your time at all. Radiology is the kind of a discipline with which even the most well trained radiologists and doctors can still have difficulty. How can we expect to use our underdeveloped skills? More importantly, why would we need to develop the skill? Emergency medicine and orthopedics are some branches of conventional medicine that will still have a place in society even when all people embrace holistic medicine. Therefore, the specialists in taking and reading X-rays, CT scans and MRIs will continue to do so. If we ever need their help, we can refer. We don't need this course at all as a part of our program.

Lab diagnosis: It's nice to know different levels and readings in the blood. It helps the naturopath who treats systems. But it is not necessary in the healing of human beings and working in harmony with the Vis. It is just a handle to get control of the situation so you can treat symptomatically, or systematically.

There is nothing wrong with the physical body in disease. It is simply a reflection of what is going on in the mind. The body, therefore, does not need to be treated as a hopeless entity, lost and malfunctional. There is nothing wrong with the thyroid in hypothyroidism. If you start giving thyroid-friendly supplements to the person's system without treating the whole of them and the cause of the thyroid's imbalance, you are giving the impression that there is something wrong with the thyroid, rather than a disharmony in the being, which manifested as a thyroid problem. In colitis, there is nothing wrong with the colon. In migraines, there is nothing wrong with the head.

In Myasthenia Gravis there isn't anything wrong with the muscles, as if they were malfunctional. The person might be attacking himself or herself. "What's the matter with you? Why aren't you perfect?" Remember that your body is playing the faithful dog. You say, "What's wrong with you?" and you attack it, it attacks itself. That is what auto-immune is. The immune system turns its cannons around and fires upon itself. In autoimmune diseases, there is nothing wrong with the immune system or its organs, like the thymus gland in M.G., which conventional medicine often surgically removes. In autoimmune disease, as soon as you give the message to your immune system to stop firing upon the self, the immune system will comply instantly.

If you feel you must look into the body to see where its levels are and diagnose laboratorily, just keep in mind that you will limit the treatment to control-based medicine, rather than helping someone heal from within. Think of the thyroid. If you discover that T4 and T3 are low, what are you going to do with that information? Are you going to start supplementing with synthetic T3 or T4? Are you going to give kelp? Where is the whole person medicine in that?

In a case of Myasthenia Gravis, if someone comes to you, undiagnosed, and they have ptosis and weak muscles, and you send their blood away and determine they have the antibodies commonly seen in Myasthenia Gravis, what are you going to do with that information? The truth is, it doesn't mean a thing to you if you are treating the whole person, because the diagnosis could be anything. You can call it, "Wasting Syndrome" ("Wei Syndrome" in Chinese medicine) if you like. You can make up a name for the condition. Whatever you call it, treating whole naturopathy, you are still going to treat the person, the individual, within his/her issues, his/her whole person, and in his/her unique pattern of imbalance and disharmony. You are not going to treat the disease. You don't have to label it and so you don't really need a lab diagnosis.

This course, therefore, would serve naturopathy better, not as a means of diagnosing disease, but as a specialty course relevant to naturopathic practice and to help students learn such things as how to read lab results to detect toxic levels of heavy metals, vitamin deficiencies, and to understand different blood markers to assess how the healing process is progressing. Yet one can also assess the healing progress by the improvement of symptoms and overall well-being, and lab diagnosis is not necessary.

Pathology and Differential Diagnosis: These courses could be treated more as reference courses, where students learn how to access information regarding the various diseases. All pathologies should be covered, enabling the naturopath to understand the language of disease, but fewer hours are necessary. The details can be left out, as they are accessible through the referencing of information, and naturopathic doctors need not focus too much in the field of disease's diagnosis and treatment. This helps deflate the fear surrounding certain diseases, as we discussed in the on diagnosis and prognosis.

The trust in the healing power of Nature and the healing process will help you see past the need to find what disease you are dealing with, which is often sought just to make you feel more secure when working with copatients. Often, when people feel sick, they also want to know what it is. What is it called? What do I have? For some reason, this often helps people feel better about the symptoms they're experiencing. "If I know what disease this is that I am suffering from, then the doctors will know what to do for me." The diagnosis is a security for fear. This is the trap we get into, because we want to dissociate ourselves from our disease, so it can just be fixed and we don't have to deal with it. The disease is not what the patients want to focus on. Healing themselves, their lives, their relationships, is what they want to focus on. The diseased state that they find themselves in is a sign that it is time that they look at how they are not living in harmony with themselves and Nature. Treat them as whole individuals, empower them to take responsibility for themselves and they will feel better. Then they won't need to have a label for their disease. Education, education, education. Doctor as teacher.

Specialty Courses: (Cardiology, dermatology, endocrinology, EENT, gastroenterology, genitourinary system, neurology, orthopedics, pulmonary, rheumatology, oncology)

These courses, with compartmentalized disease, are too close to creating a program for green MDs. The conditions and diseases that arise in the different systems are dealt with in pathology. The conditions can be referenced in the Merck Manual, on the Internet, or in other text books if necessary. All of these courses are unnecessary for the naturopathic program and will free up a lot of time for the courses that are needed for the essence of our medicine. If these courses are presented, they would serve naturopathy in the best way if examples of cases with these specific pathologies were regarded in a whole person, individualistic fashion, with the specific cause of disease addressed. It is especially important to show the students that by simply addressing and treating the cause of disease and working holistically in each case, the pathology improved, regardless of what system was affected. This sort of education is exciting for students as they get to glimpse their future helping people. They will also develop a keen sense of trust in the philosophy of our medicine by seeing that treating the cause and not the symptoms of disease or the disease itself is what ultimately benefits people.

The space created by removing unnecessary courses and cutting down the time of other courses that have been given too much importance can be used to hone our skills in counseling, homeopathy, acupuncture, hydrotherapy, herbology, nutrition, and to devote ourselves to self-development and healing. The following courses should be implemented in the core program or emphasized more:

Hydrotherapy (Nature Cure): The origins of naturopathic medicine largely involved Nature Cure. It is not emphasized enough in the program and more hours are indicated. In addition to the powerful constitutional treatment, the many simple techniques that are learned in this course, like Sitz bath, wet sock treatment, and the hydrotherapy shower, can be taught to copatients to give them tools to take care of themselves.

Homeopathy, TCM, Botanical Medicine, Nutrition: These courses make up the guts of naturopathic medicine and should be given more hours. It is a good idea to have students specialize in their preferred modalities. The first and second years could involve all students learning all of the modalities, with the third and fourth years dedicated to specializing in one or two of these courses. Rather than having a weak foundation in all of the modalities, this would hone skills in one or two of the modalities and better prepare students for practice. The overall development of the essence of our medicine is essential throughout the program –students will learn to heal themselves, develop their listening skills, their intuition, their rapport with their copatients, and recognize how to detect the cause of disease and what needs to be addressed in a person. This should be covered throughout the years regardless of what classes are taken, but especially in counseling and Physician, Heal Thyself! With the essence established as the foundation, the more skill a student has in one modality, the better. Naturopaths must then develop their modalities or modality to deal with the cause of disease and to treat each person as an individual on all levels of their being.

Counseling: When naturopathic medicine is placed back on the roots of its philosophy, counseling becomes one of the most important courses that the program can offer. It must be transformed from its present state of textbook psychology to a more dynamic, updated counseling class based in the healing paradigm. State of the art, cutting edge techniques of releasing fears, judgments, and beliefs systems including those techniques seen in spiritual counseling, hands-on-healing, psychotherapy, Option Process, Core Belief work and Gestalt therapy, for some examples, could be included. Educate students in the healing ways of counseling, which is in non-directive, non-judgmental questioning and guidance so that copatients come to their own awareness and are not simply supplied with insight by the practitioner, which is the allopathic paradigm of counseling. Make this ultra-important class worthwhile and alive; as dynamic as the twists and turns in cases where this technique is employed.

It is also essential to establish a trusting, healing environment from day one in which students feel free to share their own issues, so they can learn from each other and themselves and need not rely on the unrealistic role-playing of hired actors. This will also help carry over the process of self-healing that is essential for student growth into courses throughout the curriculum. This is established most easily when there are fewer students who know each other well enough to open up. The weaknesses and issues we have are nothing to be ashamed of. In fact, being able to share openly is part of the process of letting go that promotes healing. It sets the stage for being capable and willing to facilitate the process of opening up and sharing with copatients. If this cannot be established collectively in the college, not just in this course, but in all courses, and if we cannot learn to get past the judgment of our human weaknesses and problems, how can the students expect to do so properly in a clinical setting?

This course should receive more focus and emphasis. More hours are required to learn the various techniques of counseling that work in harmony with the Vis and to allow students to work with the techniques together at their own issues, fears, and judgments to experience this powerful process for themselves.

Physician, Heal Thyself: This is the most important course of the program. It should be given every semester of the four-year program. It will give students direct experience of the ways of healing, by first witnessing the properties, principles, effects, and the phenomena of healing on themselves. It will help students stay in balance and learn to deal with the issues that arise during the program. This is the course that brings healers into the arena to practice being what they are. It develops a student into a naturopath geared for whole person healing. It will naturally help students understand the principles of philosophy of naturopathic medicine because the principles are encountered in any healing experience.

This course will not be scholastically or intellectually challenging, which often gives students, who are entirely focused on the rational approach to learning, the impression that they need not attend. They think, "There's no exam. Why go?" Hopefully, the screening process will accept mostly students who recognize the importance of their own development for practice.

The course will be challenging on many other levels. Deep mental and emotional work is not easy. It might be simple and straightforward, but the challenge of facing one's fears, issues and pain does not come easy. It takes dedication, commitment and perseverance. This course, in healing students, heals all aspects of their lives. What they then represent and embody in the world is something more of what they truly hope to be and truly are. They carry the torch of the healing paradigm wherever they go, showing people a streak of goodness, strength, and most importantly, the great benefits of healing ourselves. In addition to that, by witnessing first hand their own healing and becoming more aware people, the students' skills in the subtle arts of our medicine, like counseling, homeopathy, and acupuncture, naturally increase.

Naturopathic medicine will not be what it is supposed to be until its students become what they are meant to be: healers, doctors who inspire and show their copatients how to heal themselves. Happy, balanced people who understand the nature of reality beyond what's found in books. To carry forward Naturopathic medicine in the best way to serve humanity, this course must be included in the program.

Included in this course will be healing from many different cultures and emerging spiritual philosophies. Learning current techniques of clearing issues, blocked energies, and imbalances through meditation, breath work, belief system counseling and clearing, and other techniques, will broaden students' awareness of various spiritual and healing modalities and will also create a better relationship with themselves. This also increases each student's repertory of skills that can be used for his/her own copatients.

As it stands now, students are immersed in courses that do not develop the skills and essence of naturopathic medicine. If students are interested in developing themselves as whole NDs, they must seek exposure to this knowledge outside of the program. It is time to reverse this situation. Let the program cover the essentials of allopathic knowledge, but be immersed in the essence of our medicine and dedicated to increasing skills and knowledge in the modalities we use. Then let students who wish to further increase their knowledge in allopathic diagnosis and treatment seek it on their own time, outside of the program.

CHAPTER 10

Whole Person Case Studies

THE CASES SHARED BELOW are to illustrate how one can think of a case in whole person terms, with some of the cause of disease exposed and discussed, and other aspects of the principles of naturopathy elaborated upon.

These example cases are illustrations of what we have discussed in this book and examples of whole person naturopathy. I share some of the protocols I chose to do and why, but the unique creativity and approach of each naturopath could express itself differently in these cases and in any case.

Case 1: Man, Age 39

He comes in for fatigue and insomnia. He has frequent recurring headaches that are dull, painful, and persistent, sometimes lasting all day. He goes to bed with his problems and worries about them. He can't stop thinking about solving his problems. Everything has to be in order, solved and neat. He won't even answer the phone sometimes because he doesn't want to know there is a problem. There are always problems in his line of business. He admits that he finds problems to worry about even when there aren't any.

Arguments with family members also disturb him a lot. It really bothers him how much his wife's mother favors her and is possessive of her. He thinks about this a lot. He plays scenarios in his head over and over. "It drives me crazy how they are so needy. That they both need each other so much. They're socially retarded." He says they are a tightly-knit family but one has to cut the umbilical cord.

He thinks his in-laws speak badly about him. They think he's jealous. That upsets him because he thinks it is likely the opposite. What he actually said about this situation is that he thinks people should be treated fairly and shouldn't show favoritism toward anyone. It's not fair, he says.

He used to work for the government and was outraged at the way they treated Blacks and Jews and some other minorities so unfairly. He took action to see it brought to justice, wrote letters, went to see superiors and was blown away to find the depth of the problem. People didn't care and were prejudiced even in the highest positions of the government. He was really enraged. He still thinks about it but hasn't really done anything. "Injustice really fires me up." He has lost sleep over it. "I should have said this. I should have said that."

He lives in Quebec, a French-Canadian province. He isn't French. He is a minority, not visible, but a minority through language. He thinks the French people discriminate against him when they discover he isn't French. He feels persecuted and doesn't like or trust the French. He thinks they're all prejudiced.

He says that his brother was favoured as a child, although he is just as intelligent as his brother. His father was very hard on him, forcing him to learn math when he was three. Needed him to be perfect in his father's way. He wouldn't do it so his father stopped giving him any compliments and encouragement as he went through school. This created a gap between how his father treated his brother and himself. It wasn't fair, he felt. "I'm just as intelligent as my brother." His response was to either do really well or fail completely. He also became a rebel, a trouble maker and a delinquent. He would get back at people who treated him unfairly. He always liked the excitement of studying material that was way ahead of his grade, like high school chemistry in elementary school. He read "The Communist Manifesto' in grade three.

Discussion of Case 1

In many cases, you might not see the theme that governs a person's entire life. So you help a person with each issue as it comes up, like anger and fear of certain situations, insecurities triggered by certain people, until many of their issues, fears and choices coalesce into the central theme of his/her life which has kept him/her bound, stressed out, unhappy, and unhealthy. In this case, his feeling inside is of being treated unfairly, unjustly. It bothers him that his wife's mother favours her daughter over him because it is a reenactment of the treatment he got from his father. His brother was favoured because he complied with his father's demands. What this man kept telling me, perhaps not even aware of what he was trying to say, is that he was just as intelligent as his brother but refused to do what his father told him, so he was treated unfairly. Who wants to be forced to learn math at the age of three? His choice to be himself resulted in his father's withdrawal of his love and acceptance (no longer complimenting him). He continued to live his life with this inherent feeling of not being accepted, not being good enough. Inside, he always wanted his father's approval even if he had rebelled against his father's control. His reaction to this was that IT wasn't fair. As a result, he adopted a belief system that life isn't fair, which includes people not being fair, family, friendships, etc. That is why he couldn't tolerate any injustice anywhere and also felt as if he was being persecuted by people and treated unfairly. This is his projection of his own reality onto life. It is true that some people are prejudiced. But to live life as if everyone is prejudiced, is a projection of a belief system and limits one to a negative and lesser reality.

This man's life was a series of extremes—trying hard to be perfect in everything (incessant worry about how to solve problems, reading advanced materials to have the upper hand in intelligence) and completely rebelling by failing or being a delinquent. His reactions were always to fight against the things that reminded him of his father's favoritism toward his brother and lack of love toward himself. What is also very important to understand in this case is that even though he rebelled and rejected his father's control, since his father didn't give him love as a result, this man was still seeking the love and acceptance of his father. This need to get the love and acceptance from a man who wouldn't show it and needed everything to be perfect himself resulted in the symptom of being a perfectionist—of needing to solve problems, of being on top of things, having everything in control. It was a round-about and indirect way of saying, "Look Dad, I am okay too. I have everything in control and ordered. I am successful and on the ball. You can love me now, you know."

Imagine the immense amount of emotion that can build up in people who feel they are being treated unfairly and not loved for who they are, not only by the people of their country, but by their loved ones. They are constantly on guard for this injustice. Being on guard does not promote health. Even though his pathology did not extend beyond headaches, insomnia and fatigue, he is not at peace with himself or the world. He is in a state of dis-ease. He worries constantly because he thinks he has to be perfect (learned from his father) and that he isn't good enough. There might be issues with the mother too, but they didn't present themselves.

When you worry, you become stressed out. You hurry and are not at peace. This stimulates the sympathetic nervous system which suppresses the immune system, stresses out the kidneys and the heart, and keeps the digestive and elimination system acting suboptimally, since they act best at rest and in parasympathetic mode, which is where healing occurs. All cases present stress in different manners. This case's stress is the stress of being treated unfairly. And being treated unfairly, you learn, is because you think like an individual, you have your own head on your shoulders and will not change who you are just to get someone's love, even though you long for it all along. The real feeling might be, "If I am true to myself, and just be myself, others whom I love and care for will not love me.

They will treat me unfairly." The response is to rebel, to fight against that which treats you unfairly. This is why this person is dis-eased. He is always fighting.

To help people make the connections between all the issues in their lives is very valuable. To help them understand the theme of their life is priceless, especially if you facilitate their awareness and lead them to their own discovery. A very good way to do it is through non-directive counseling. Non-directive is the most effective way because the awareness comes from within the copatient, not from the doctor. Counseling that is directional based, by the physician offering advice, is allopathic in nature. It is using the doctor as the source of the healing. It doesn't work as well, and sometimes not at all. The doctor or counselor will say, "You are fighting injustice because your father treated you unfairly," and the copatient will say, "Yes this is true," and it will not penetrate unless they discover it for themselves. It can even cause a real internal frustration to know it on a mental level yet not have the awareness penetrate into feeling it on an intuitive level. When it does penetrate intuitively so people get a real sense of just how deep and true that awareness is for them, the healing has already begun.

Diet is indicated in every case. In this case especially, because he was most tired after his lunches, which were comprised of cold-cut sandwiches made on wheat bread. The switch to kamut, spelt, rice, or other non-gluten grains for his lunch bread would help him get through the day, as would eating meat of better quality. Homeopathy is a good idea in any case. It is one of the most powerful tools we have to carry out all the principles of our naturopathic philosophy. You can treat the whole person and the individual homeopathically, matching their issues, fears, judgments and belief systems to a substance in nature that covers their totality and their essence. The healing ultimately occurs from within them, in harmony with the healing powers of nature, when they see themselves (consciously or subconsciously) reflected by the remedy that is so similar to them. In this case, I gave him Mercurius. (He had some other symptoms that are typical of the paradoxical nature of Mercurius. For instance, he said he didn't believe in God yet he prayed every day.)

In the approach of whole person healing, this person's healing process will not occur overnight because it involves the reprogramming of beliefs and emotional responses that have been embedded since childhood. Nevertheless, the case did improve. He wasn't sure if it was the remedy. He thought what helped him the most was realizing how hard he had been trying to be perfect and he was able to make the connection that it was trying to be perfect, trying to please his father. When he realized that his dad wasn't ever going to accept him and that he needed to accept himself, he stopped worrying a lot.

Accepting oneself is an invaluable exercise. You have to live with yourself constantly. Your foundation must therefore be based 100%, totally and completely upon your own acceptance, not someone else's. In this case, his father loved him conditionally, which is not the best way of raising a child. But so many people were raised in this fashion because of the challenge that bringing up children posed upon the parents, and how it triggered their own issues and fears. Our healing paths therefore must take us in to heal the realm where we still live attached to our parents, yearning for their love and acceptance of who we really are and not what they think we should be. We must go there and detach, finding our own self again, accepting ourselves totally without the need for anyone else's approval.

What helped this man the most? Was it the counseling, the homeopathy, the diet changes, or was it just the commitment of going to see somebody for his health? I don't know. It doesn't really matter to me. The medicine is not a series of compartments of modalities. As long as the ultimate goal is the health and well-being of the person, and the selected treatments are all aligned with whole person, treating-the-cause naturopathy, it is the totality of the modalities that ultimately works.

Case 2: Woman, Age 24

She comes to see me for many problems and with what seems like much deep-seated pathology. She is having neurological problems like uncontrollable shaking, uncontrollable laughter and epileptic-like seizures that involve trembling and inability to speak. She has had all the tests and they couldn't find anything wrong with her. She is on a lot of meds for the neurological symptoms and also for depression and for type I diabetes and diabetic neuropathy. She also has a lot of mood swings.

She has type I diabetes, which she tells me she had created to keep her father from sexually, emotionally and physically abusing her. She says it worked. He stopped once she was really sick. He called her all sorts of names. Her oldest memory, amazingly, was of an argument her parents had a few days after she was born where her father said he didn't want a girl and told the mother to "get rid of her." During the time he was abusing her, he bribed her emotionally, telling her that he wouldn't love her or he'd hurt her sisters if she told anyone. She couldn't speak about it to anyone.

She is disgusted with a lot of people. At men, she says, for being such idiots and at her father for the obvious. At her mother for pretending everything was okay and letting it happen, not stopping it. "You should have protected me!!!" She is angry at society because it is so aggravating and she especially hates "New Money" because everyone listens to those people just because they are rich. No one really listens to her, she says, because of her socio-economic situation, and she has such important things to say.

She loves animals because "We communicate really well." They understand each other. As a child, when she felt nobody understood her in her family, she would run out to the barn and sleep curled up on her horse.

In relationships with men, she feels needy. She needs to be held, and told how wonderful she is. It was too much for her boyfriend. It pushed him away.

The times she has laughing attacks or seizures come when she isn't understood by people, doctors, her friends, her parents. She feels completely frustrated and then calls them names, and then laughs uncontrollably or shakes or is unable to say anything at all. Her expression also splits into the extremes of very aggressive and abusive, cornering people and letting them know what she was feeling, to not saying a word, feeling unheard and misunderstood and being extremely frustrated.

She is incredibly intelligent and uses her intellect to rationalize and control her feelings, protecting her from the inner pain. As soon as she gets close to the feelings of pain, she says, "Ah but that isn't relevant," dismissing her feelings. She starts to become witty, which leads to expressions of anger at everyone not understanding her and being so stupid. Then she laughs. She is aware of this control over her emotions but is terrified of facing the feelings. She says she hasn't let herself feel for as long as she can remember. She prides herself on the fact that she is well read and has a snappy answer for everything, but she can also be made to feel stupid. She knows and understands the connection of becoming witty and cerebral to avoid her feelings. Overall, she is very aware of why and how she is ill.

She has been bleeding vaginally for one year since she had a miscarriage the previous year. She is grief-stricken from losing the baby. She also experienced a lot of pain associated with the diabetic neuropathy. She was on drugs for that too. She had a pattern of four days diarrhea then four days of constipation.

Discussion of Case 2

At first, with so much going on and so many symptoms, this case can seem overwhelming. Can you imagine the allopathic approach? It would involve addressing the troubles with her nervous system. It would involve treating the diabetes, and the depression and the bleeding. It would cost a fortune in lab tests and supplements. She had no money. No matter how wealthy a person is, I always rejoice at the incredible cost-effectiveness of whole person naturopathy. We have the ability to work with the healing power of Nature without relying on numerous outside substances. The allopathic approach in this case would have been a great waste of time, because all of her problems stemmed from one issue, and addressing that, the whole case began to clear up.

Fortunately this case provided a clear-cut theme, so the path of whole person naturopathy was laid out for us. She felt unheard and hurt. Hurt leads to pain. Pain to anger. It all came from her father threatening her to not say anything "or else" and her mother not picking up on her other ways of indirectly crying out for help—outbursts, temper tantrums, getting ill. When peoples' expression outlets are plugged up, they learn to rely on others to sense that something is wrong with them. In fact, they need it, just as this child needed her mother to see what she was going through. This led to hatred of her mother who should have gotten it, and following that, hatred of all people who didn't listen to or understand her. She said she would have problems with communication in her relationship with her boyfriend and her friends. If she was upset, she would become silent and upset and expect them to figure out what was going on. If they didn't, she'd get mad and disgusted with them and think they were stupid.

She didn't feel the right to express her unhappiness or anger directly. Her healing came from removing the block over her throat energetic system/chakra, over the outlet to express what was not right in her life and stepping her rational mind out of the way so that she could reconnect with those emotions she has suppressed for so long.

Suppressed emotions cause sickness. The Three Treasures of this case shows us that the mind wasn't allowing the Qi to flow, (this is her blocking her emotions), and the body wasn't getting the nourishment from the blood, because the flow of her blood was reflecting the suppressed flow of her Qi. This is how she got sick. There was nothing wrong with her neurological system giving her convulsions, nor her uterus for bleeding. The lab diagnoses and all the other tests showed nothing wrong. Even if they had shown an abnormality, it would be the body reflecting the inner disharmony of this woman's mind, emotions and her relationship to herself and her environment. In this case, she was grieving on all levels of her being and didn't know how to express it or come to terms with it, so her energy was blocked. In response, her nervous system acted out of sorts and out of control to express how chaotically she was feeling inside. Her uterus was weeping blood in expression of her grief. Her anger and frustration at not being heard was so much she couldn't take it, so she'd laugh uncontrollably or shake. Her blockage of expression manifested obviously as the moments when the seizures wouldn't let her speak at all.

The causes of disease in this case and the last stem from the mental emotional sphere. Addressing this cause by facing it and clearing it, we allow the healing power of Nature to do Her work. This is whole person medicine. This is doctor as teacher. This is treating each person as an individual. This is the gift that the art and science of naturopathic medicine offers the world, because our understanding encompasses so many angles on our health. It is our view of reality and the choices we subsequently make from our childhood experiences that cause us to become out of accord with our inner balance, our vital force. Even for a young child who adopts patterns from parents or seems to decide things that are beyond its young awareness, the child still is actively choosing—these beliefs and behaviours. The child usually does it for love. In Case 1, the young boy wanted his father's recognition and acceptance. He could live his whole life wishing for it and trying to control his life around getting this acceptance from his dad and all those people who remind him in any way of his dad—father figures, organizations, groups of people. In Case 2, the choice this girl makes is forced upon her by the situation. She nevertheless holds onto it as she grows, by her own will, perhaps waiting for someone who loves her to hear her pleas for help. She could have done that for the rest of her life if she didn't choose to heal herself.

Mistreated children often take personal blame, continuing to believe that there must be something wrong with them because their parents treat them with so little love. This woman had a deep feeling of having something wrong with her, and was looking for acceptance and love from her father, who continued to treat her terribly. It is like that in any situation of such extremes of control or abuse. The controller feeds on the other's need to gain acceptance. Often, the controlling person's, or the abuser's, belief is that if they were to give love freely without needing anything in return, then they wouldn't be needed anymore. As long as they withhold any sort of love and affection, their child remains dependent, always waiting for an expression of care and warmth.

The empowerment that comes from each of these cases releasing these childhood beliefs and patterns of behaviour is invaluable for health and well-being. The power to do so comes only from them. One cannot make them see it or make them want to change their minds. When they are ready, they will make the shift themselves and the explosion of vitality that results from the shedding of childhood delusions and suppressed pain will have come about by their *own* wills. That makes the whole difference.

Case 2 called for any form of treatment that could help this young woman to feel her emotions and deal with the pain from her childhood. The path of healing is the journey we take to return to the state we existed in before we were hurt, and before our reality went from harmony to dissonance. It is not always easy. It requires the support of a loving, understanding healer to encourage the facing of and letting go of pain, and to clear the belief systems that we hold on to our entire lives. Counseling is a wonderful way to help people come to these awarenesses and provides that support for people to explore what they believe about themselves and about life that is making them unhappy and unhealthy.

I gave the woman Ignatia homeopathically, which treated her totality and the theme of her life—feeling unheard, misunderstood and hurt. She hated being on the drugs she was on so we stopped those completely after several weeks. She didn't need them anyway. After six weeks, the seizures were reduced to mild shaking only at night and the laughter fits and loss of speech stopped altogether, as did the vaginal bleeding. She felt better emotionally and didn't need to take the antidepressants she had been on. (Another possible remedy for this case could have been Hepar Sulph or Calc. Sulph.—the theme of not being supported and protected in the place of love, of being misunderstood, and the great amounts of anger. She also told me that she had a fear of things catching fire, one of the keynotes of Hepar sulph. This could be an even deeper remedy for her).

It is likely that this case benefited quite a lot from the remedy. But she had come to the realization, through the history taking and counseling, that she felt misunderstood and unheard throughout her life and it was this that brought on the seizures and neurological phenomena. She said she was able to dig deeply because she felt totally and completely comfortable allowing her immensely bottled up emotions to be expressed. I gave her the space to be angry, disgusted, sad, and insecure. This is simply a blank state of being that one goes into, being non-judgmental and trusting totally in the process that the copatient needs to go through. Do I know for sure which element brought about the healing? No. She understood the importance of expressing herself better and was doing so. That is why she was healthier. It just so "happens" that a lot of her symptoms also went away too. That's what happens when the whole person is treated along with the cause.

CHAPTER 11

Love in Medicine

The main reason for healing is love.

—Paracelsus

THERE IS ONE THING that brought us into the world and when we die, we will return to it. It is the basis and foundation of the major religions of the world. When we are born into a world without it, it makes us sick, and we become even sicker when we do not impart it and share it in our lives. When dealing with the subject of health, it is the number one issue responsible for the health of our planet, whether it is the absence of it that creates misery, suffering, and dis-ease, or the presence of it bringing peace, harmony and well-being. That one thing is love.

When children are brought up in a family that is devoid of love, they become sick. Their view of reality is distorted. They do not understand how the world can be a happy place, where people help each other and look out for each other. Their reality becomes skewed and when this occurs, they are dis-eased. Even if they never manifest disease on a physical level, they are imbalanced and ill because they are not experiencing or witnessing the world as it could be; joyous, caring, and loving, but as they learned it to be; loveless and cold.

Since naturopathic doctors are not just responsible for treating the physical manifestation of disease, we therefore must understand the importance of love within our profession. Love is something that is impossible to convey to another through rational terms. It is not possible to even directly communicate its essence, its qualities.

Science will never reproduce or even remotely understand the fullness and depth of love.

> Man can try to name love, showering upon it all the names at his command, and still he will involve himself in endless self-deceptions. If he posses a grain of wisdom, he will lay down his arms and name the unknown by the more unknown... by the name of God.
>
> —Carl G. Jung

God is one name that we have given for that divine force that inhabits all places and encompasses all things. It is the Source of life and the place we go to when we die. Love is of the very same essence, and being vital and crucial to life, yet at the same time unknown, we cannot ever put our finger on it. Love is the healing power of Nature, which is something also that we can never fully grasp or define. What we can all do is embody love in our practices. By perceiving the people that come into our lives seeking our care and guidance, we place our relationships with our copatients into the proper space where we allow the healing power of Nature to work through us. Even if one has few or no skills as a physician, a naturopath whose practice is imbibed with love is a good naturopath. Just by their presence and their state of being, they will have a positive influence on the well-being of their copatients.

Love is our natural state. It is a state that we experience and share when we are healthy and happy. It is more than just the romantic notion of it that we think of in relationship between lovers. Love is kindness, caring, and compassion. It is the courage you need to be true to who you are. It is the faith to know that what you are doing is good even when you're surrounded by opposition. Love is the default. When we get become dis-eased, we experience and express a nature other than how we were created to be. When we go upon the path of healing, it is to return to the state where love teaches us that we are okay, and even better than that, we are good and the world where we live is as well. When we live in such a reality, our actions reflect kindly upon the world, enhancing its content with our contribution that comes from the goodness of our hearts. This is the natural path that a naturopath does well to walk upon.

Love is the single most important factor in the healing of humanity. It is the strength and wisdom that is brought into a sick situation to make it better. It is the miraculous energy that finds a solution to impossibly corrupt situations and to severely ill conditions. Remembering how to love is returning to a place where we naturally exist in a perfectly healthy state.

Since naturopaths are whole person healers, we are also whole life healers, taking into account everything that can have a positive influence on our health and the well-being of our planet. Naturopaths and other healers will eventually and naturally spill into every aspect of life and into every niche of society that needs healing. You will see NDs working to heal our limiting education system and our sick hospitals. You will see NDs and other healers doling out their doses of love for homeless people and street kids. When people rise into positions of power, they have a great influence on many people's lives. If they are not well and are not in, when their reality is not one of love, then they are not going to be able to create healthy situations for the people they govern. Therefore, you will see naturopaths finding their way into these positions to heal not only the body of people who sit in government, but also the mind of the government that is misaligned with its true purpose.

The left brain and the rational mind, the mind that sits solely in scientific evidence, is uncomfortable speaking of love. It calls it "airy fairy" and belittles the importance of it because it feels threatened by love's immense healing power. The reason it feels threatened is because the healing power of the heart threatens its very existence. It knows that in a space that is filled with love, people will not employ its use, because they have no need.

What happens to the magic of a loving moment, sharing an embrace, a magical healing connection with another, when you step up into your brain to think about it? The magic is gone. And the converse is true. When you step into the space of the heart, no longer does the voice of the defined and rational left brain order you around. Naturally, it will want to scoff at the idea of love being the most important factor in medicine and healing. What would happen to the importance of all of its knowledge and learning, everything that gives it existence, if it were to accept the all-encompassing healing power of love, which is not something you can learn, but something that exists inherently in who you are?

The rational mind jumps in to control in situations of fear and pain. Insomuch as a person is unwell or afraid, he/she will be proportionally rational. In my practice, I see the switch from heartfelt feelings to the rational mind when people begin to explore their painful spots. They will share freely until they get deep into their pain where they will begin to make excuses or attempt to rationalize everything. The rational mind puts the brakes onto the whole process of being truthful with one's feelings. Instead of being honest and facing the hurt in those places where we are not connected to love in order to move through the pain to the other side, the rational mind might say something like, "What's the point? I've been this way my whole life. I cannot change." In other cases, instead of trusting one's gut feeling to leave an unhealthy relationship, the rational mind will state, "Maybe it's just me that can't deal with things."

What is the number one killer in North America? It is disease of the heart because so many people switch off their hearts to live in their heads. As soon as this happens, they start to die inside. It is only a matter of time until their heart says, "I've had it! I give up," because it isn't allowed to rejoice on waking for what it has to do during the day. It isn't allowed to celebrate a person's life choices because the person isn't doing what they love. It chose to uphold those beliefs that were adopted at some point from other people, and not one's own innermost longing.

The reality of love always shows you the solution to unhealthy situations and how to find your way out of the maze of disease. Following the way of love is to find abundance of vitality, ecstasy of being, and Heaven on Earth. Imagine the effects of living your entire life not according to what you love but according to what you think you must. "Where will I get the money?" "What will Mom and Dad think?" "What if I fail?" "What will this look like to others?" The difference of living what you love versus living what you think you should or running from your fears is immense. In chronic disease, it is the difference between sickness and health.

As naturopaths, we face the challenge of doing what we love versus doing all those things we think we should to be recognized. We know the importance of living what we love in our education and our profession. Letting love trickle into our naturopathic education will yield a healthy program with happy, effective naturopathic doctors. We know the importance of love in our lives, when we greet people on the street or at the supermarket. And since love is a natural state that bubbles out of people when they are being true to themselves, and since being untrue to oneself is to be dis-eased, we recognize the importance of doing everything that we can to be true to the nature of our medicine. We can spot the importance of switching from evidence-based medicine to the simplicity of an empirical medicine that directly and intuitively understands the principles of healing without proof. We especially recognize the necessity of the 7th philosophy of naturopathic medicine to heal ourselves, because in doing so, in becoming healed, we are happy. When you are happy, you can live who you are and constantly rediscover that your whole world revolves around love. What you live and embody, you have no difficulty or hesitation sharing outwardly with the public. Thus we know the importance of freely speaking, showing, and sharing love in the corridors of our colleges, amongst our peers, family and friends, and of course with our copatients.

CHAPTER 12

Trusting the Healing Process

IN OUR PRACTICES, and in the teaching environment of our colleges, it is very important to trust the healing process. This involves knowing that we are capable of helping people and that the modalities we use are effective. It is having faith in the philosophy of our medicine, knowing that it works. The simplicity of whole person naturopathy, baffling as it is to the complicated mind, is something that we can trust in to allow the healing process to take place.

A lot of the trust comes from seeing how the process of healing has worked for you. Even if you don't have a physical disease, you might have anxiety, fears, and other stresses. You might have trouble going to the bathroom or have little energy. You can heal yourself in the ways in which you are not happy and living life the way you truly want to. In so doing, you trust the process of healing, having witnessed the great sense of freedom, the empowerment of being yourself and all the energy and vitality for your body that comes from living that way.

Understanding the relationship between the Mind, Qi, and Blood, or the mind, emotions and the physical body, as discussed in chapter 3, will greatly help you know how to address the cause and have trust in the healing that results from doing so.

We must also know that healing often occurs gradually and does not always occur instantly. The potential for a rapid and complete cure does exist, but the potential is subject to the individual's willingness to let it happen by stepping into the realm of well-being. Usually, healing takes place slowly, like the slow growth, budding, and opening of a flower. Over time, if copatients were to look back, they will see the great difference over the months in their overall health and well-being. But during the potentially slow process of healing and subtle shifts in outlooks on life and in energy levels, the healing process can seem undetectable. It is most certainly happening, but the lack of trust that can make you want to jump in to speeds things up, can throw the train off its tracks.

The approach of allopathic medicine is to give drugs or surgically remove things that hurt and that do not function properly. This often elicits immediate results and the patient begins to feel better right away, which many people have gotten used to and expect in all forms of medicine. But this is not a way of medicine that helps a person in the long run. Naturopaths, therefore, must take the time to paint the picture of holistic medicine and to explain that, simply surgically removing parts or giving drugs to control symptoms involves no healing.

In some cases, it is important to walk down the allopathic road, which is a subjective decision made by the physician. Other times, based in our insecurity or our need to feel effective, we wish to give a form of treatment that makes people feel better right away. This is a way in which fear can creep into practice, which comes along with insecurity, and the desire to take responsibility for the copatient's health. Our fears and insecurities can make a case that could be treated holistically and naturopathically seem as if it should be treated allopathically. It is the projection of our own worries onto our copatients and is not trusting the healing process.

If someone has been in chronic pain, or has had some chronic condition, he/she is used to it. You don't have to rescue these copatients from their pain or condition just because they came to you seeking relief. You can heal their whole person. If you treat holistically, the pain will rapidly or gradually go away. And it won't come back worse when you take the copatients off whatever substance you put them on to mask the pain. They will have been healed from within. The condition might go away slowly. Instead of receiving relief in a day, the condition might start getting better right away but will not be noticeably better for days, weeks, or even months. Can you accept that and feel confident and comfortable explaining this to your copatients? When you accept the fact that healing can be subtle and slow, you will have a easier time walking within the philosophy of our medicine.

The secret is in trusting the healing process. Your confidence and clarity will convey the necessary trust in the process with which your copatients need to align themselves. If you panic because your need to be effective makes you rescue the copatients from their symptoms and issues, you are doing them a disservice. It might feel right, but it is actually trusting the process of healing, even if it allows the lingering of certain symptoms, that is the most effective. By trusting the slow rhythms of Nature, you see there is a lot of room to operate. You might take a course of action that initially yields few results. In seeing that, you understand your copatient to a greater degree and can choose a course of action that is better aligned to bring them through the cause of their disease.

People make choices their entire lives that affect their health. You are helping them heal by facilitating the reversal of mental, emotional, physical or spiritual processes that have been harming them for a long time. Sometimes these choices have been affecting their health for several decades. This takes time to change. The cascade of mind affecting Qi affecting blood and body also takes some time to reverse. A very good thought to have is knowing that your copatients will begin to get better *as soon as* you address the cause.

Trust is a vital ingredient that can make a case when it is present, and break another when it is absent. Any insecurity and lack of trust on our parts can lead to wanting immediate results so that our copatients won't abandon us. "Why is it taking so long?!?' We project these thoughts upon them. We think they're thinking that. Sometimes they are. They also might not be needing immediate results and can be trusting in you and the process. The relationship that you establish with your copatient, after that first visit, or perhaps further on, might be enough for that person to trust you and take the chance of experiencing his/her healing process with you. Which of the two possible thinking processes would you like to focus on? Never assume that your copatients are expecting immediate results. It might just be your own projection.

If someone has suffered for a long time and has the idea that it should go away right away, he/she is not claiming responsibility for his/her health. The naturopath's goal, having been through his/her own healing process and knowing how life is intimately intertwined with health, is not simply to make people feel better in relation to their symptoms and disease but to also help their copatients understand the relationship between their health, well-being and how they are living their lives. This is "Doctor as teacher." If your goal is just to correct disease, then you fail to fulfill your role as teacher, guide, and example. You forget to work with people on all levels of their being.

What can also increase the difficulty of helping someone understand the subtleties of the healing process is that the healing process can give the impression that things are getting worse before they get better. It is not entirely accurate to call this an aggravation, and in understanding properly, we can convey what is actually happening to better help people through the process.

People can get sick from suppressing their anger, due to the whole cascade that suppression of Qi and emotion causes. They usually suppress anger because they grew up judging its expression as something bad. When they start to heal, the anger they have suppressed will surface for them to deal with. All the effects that this suppressed anger has had on the internal organs, muscles and tissues must be released once the blocking process has been reversed. Allowing the unnatural resistance of the expression of certain judged emotions and feelings to clear themselves is a very empowering phenomenon. This is the same for anything that is suppressed. The healing occurs once the judgment of that suppressed emotion is released. Whatever the emotion may be, it will not feel pleasant to face the very thing they have judged as bad and that they haven't allowed themselves to experience. But to heal, this must happen. They must let the suppressed energies and states of being resume their flow or there will be no lasting healing and sense of well-being.

The secret to understand is that the symptoms might seem to get worse, when they are actually getting better. Things are coming unstuck. That which was frozen dethaws. That which has not been allowed to be, is being. If all your life you judged the expression of anger and suppressed it, and when healing begins the anger starts to surface, of course you might think it is getting worse. But it is not. And understanding this, we can help our copatients go through the waterfall of emotion to the cave of wonders on the other side.

People also get ill when they run around anxiously trying to fulfill their duty by serving everyone and not themselves. This pattern of behaviour can come from a person's belief that they don't matter and the only way they can count is to be helpful to everyone. It will feel highly unnatural to them, even wrong, and can bring up a lot of guilt, when they include themselves in the equation. When they start saying NO to people, it can be difficult. They grew up with the belief that they didn't count. This belief could have come from the copatient's parents. It can feel wrong, even bad, when the healing brings them to care for themselves. They are flying in the face of what they learned from those whom they loved. They might even resist initially. The healing will feel uncomfortable, like being dragged along the ground away from where you grew up. But a person must confront the beliefs that have caused them to become diseased. It is not always easy but it is necessary. The process is in the direction of improvement, not in the wrong direction, as the word aggravation can sometimes imply.

> People with heart problems and burnout had oriented their priorities around their work. Some of these people had to learn to trust others and delegate authority. Their healing process included asking themselves why they needed to control so much. Usually they found they didn't feel safe without the control. They lived by will rather than by their heart.
>
> —Barbara Ann Brennan from *Light Emerging*, p. 81

In a case of a person who needs to trust others more, the letting go of control can feel threatening. But they must let go to find the balance that is their healing.

People can feel as if they are getting worse even when all signs suggest they are getting better. Their pulse is stronger, their eyes are brighter, they have more energy, are sleeping better, are moving their bowels better, yet they continue to feel no better, perhaps even worse, than before. It is a very strange phenomenon. You can even ask them about their specific symptoms and they will tell you they have gotten somewhat better—then why do they feel as if they are getting worse or have not improved at all? It is because, due to their increase in vitality and well-being, they are suddenly more sensitive to the ways in which they are still unbalanced and out of harmony. Healing increases sensitivity on all levels. It is as if their entire organism, by beginning the healing process, has suddenly come awake to protest the remainder of any dis-ease within them and the new sensitivity within them is now that much more aware of what is not right within.

> Most of the time, people experience an immediate internal improvement. Then later, patients seem to regress. At this point, they often questioned the treatment. Many times they thought they were worse off than before they came. Their energy fields clearly indicated that they were indeed better. The imbalances in their fields were much less; their organs

were functioning better. Despite their more balanced fields, however, they were experiencing the imbalances they had more acutely. What was happening was they were becoming less tolerant of imbalances that at one time felt 'normal' to them. In short, they were in better health.
—Barbara Ann Brennan, *Light Emerging*, p. 83

Sometimes healing is painful and difficult, but it doesn't have to be. Healing is most often a pleasurable experience, full of cathartic release and joyous liberation. The potential for us to go directly into a healed space is always there. What usually makes it hard is our resistance to step into the healed space. We clutch onto the past, holding onto our pain for dear life, as if to let it go will bring it crashing down upon us again.

What is also interesting is that the very thing which people resist from feeling, which they have judged as bad, will actually appear to them as something wonderful once they have crossed into a healthy space and are seeing things from "the other side," where they are being truer to themselves, having released their pain and no longer needing to live in their illusions.

Out of your vulnerabilities will come your strength."
—Sigmund Freud

When the expression of anger is in balance and expressed during the times it is necessary, it will be a joy, not something to sweep under the carpet. Saying NO and taking time for the self will bring a great sense of strength and security, not a deep feeling of guilt. Delegating authority, something that was always avoided, will bring a true sense of power, not power over people, as it needed to be previously, but a power coming from the infinite well inside that needs nothing from the outside to feel strong and in control.

Trust in the process. It might be a good idea to explain that the process can take some time. It helps people understand who have always stepped aside from their own relationship to their health and expected immediate results. Know that as soon as you start to work together, the improvement begins. If people need to be cured instantly, explain that the process takes time. You are doing a service by explaining the difference between the allopathic paradigm and the paradigm of healing. Don't regurgitate the principles of our philosophy as they appear on all the flyers we hand out as if that will clarify anything. Explain how we are all responsible for our health, how our choices affect our lives, how our minds and bodies are connected as one, how treating the root is deeper and longer acting than just treating the branches.

With any new copatient I always say the following, "I am a naturopathic doctor. What that means is that I work to help people take responsibility for their health." Or you can say, "I encourage people to take responsibility for their health." This initial statement is a powerful way of beginning the healing relationship. Sometimes people will say, "Oh yes, I know that. I do take responsibility for my health." That is refreshing, and knowing it, it frees you to work in a much deeper and healthier way than if you pursue the co-dependant doctor-as-rescuer role. If someone doesn't know what you're talking about, or if it scares them, that is the best time to explain very patiently and in great detail what you mean. Once you have explained this, if they do come to see you, you have already established the proper foundation for the treatment. The responsibility for their health is in their hands, not yours.

I have never scared new copatients away when I have said this opening statement. But what I had done, even if they did not initially understand, was to plant a seed in their minds that grew as the healing continued, until they got it and saw their power to heal themselves. Then they visited me less and less frequently. This statement also allows you to refer back to it to remind your copatients of what they agreed to do if they start slipping into "Fix me. You're the doctor." It also establishes a relationship where you are not the doctor standing above your patients, but working with them as an co-equals, both knowing that we are all responsible for our own health.

Because you are not trying to be like God with your patient, you can be yourself, sharing heart to heart, as one would with a friend. This is an equal relationship, a co-relationship with your co-patient. Enthusiastically describe the benefits of your own healing process, the ups and downs, the challenges, and the triumphs. You do not have to have that professionally delineated relationship where you are a sealed vault and the copatient knows absolutely nothing about you. You are no different from them, and no better. You are just facilitating their health. You are really only guiding them to heal themselves. You can help them be who they are by being yourself. They will respect you for that and it will inspire them to be themselves too. One who does not open his/her heart, one who doesn't connect on the level of the heart and bring the relationship into the personal, one who must be the perfect image of unemotional professionalism, does not encourage another's freedom to share his/her own inner self. In being yourself, trusting the healing process, and by keeping an equal relationship, you will facilitate your copatient's move into health and well-being.

Conclusion

When someone has little potential for greatness and lives a mediocre existence, no one pays them too much attention. All accept them for who they are. But if someone has a great potential, and they live in mediocrity, an outcry ensues, because a great error is occurring: someone is not existing as they were created to be.

Our profession is destined for greatness. That greatness is the fulfillment of a service to bring greater health and awareness to this planet. It is the role we have in bringing medicine to a gentler and deeper place where it affects health on all levels. Through all our work with our copatients, we impact the world by setting people free to be themselves; healthier, happier, and more at peace. Through our example and our education, we help people remember that they are responsible for their health, and that their well-being is not separated from the other dimensions of their life.

The task that naturopathic medicine faces involves many challenges. It is almost impossible for the individuals of this profession to carry out this task by themselves, for they will only make little splashes here and there, especially if the profession remains divided. We must unite under the flag of our philosophy and the healing paradigm, so that our strength in numbers creates a sea of purpose, with the voices we need to be heard and the momentum we require to get our engines running in service of our roots and essence.

For all the naturopaths out in the field who have always understood the importance of embracing the healing paradigm in naturopathic medicine, you are required to take a seat in the foundation of our profession in its curriculum, aligned with its philosophy. You are needed now to lead courses such as "Physician, Heal Thyself!" and all other courses that bring the light of our medicine to our colleges as an example for the student naturopaths. You are essential to tip the tide in the right direction so that our students will have what they need to embrace our philosophy, and also learn *how* to embrace it. You have a place in the clinic, to help clinicians blossom into the whole NDs they will be and to encourage them to trust themselves and their unique healing gifts.

For all who are associated with the profession, whether it be as administrators, presidents, deans and curriculum designers, counsel members, security guards, or professional suppliers, all of your roles are crucial for the state of our profession. If you have the insight to know that attempting to gain accreditation by emulating the established science of evidence-based medicine will ultimately devastate the essence of our profession, then unite with those of like mind and make changes in this wonderful healing profession to align it with the philosophy that provides its unique identity. Have trust that we can find a way of establishing ourselves as credible and safe with the law-makers and governments of our countries while being true to our medicine. Understand that the choices we have made in attempts to appear credible and professional are adopted from other ways of thinking. Our role and philosophy are different from other professions. We are Nature doctors. That means that the guidance and expression of our medicine comes from Nature. The way this should therefore express itself is quite different from many other professions that have their foundations in science and that only step into the places on the map where science has trodden. Keep in mind also when making decisions, establishing rules and regulations, and seeking accreditation, that we should not self-regulate in ways that compromise the heart and soul of our medicine.

What we require now are people with the clear vision of naturopathic medicine to work for the profession. The principles of our philosophy do not only permeate the world of healing, but all territories of life, because they work in harmony with Nature. And so you will find healing comes to *your* life when you work toward healing the profession. The favour that will shine down on you will be unmistakable, because you will be serving all of humanity by helping this profession stand on its proper roots.

Our political correctness will not serve us if we allow our education to lack in whole person naturopathy. Our political correctness will lead to the obsolescence of our profession if we do not face the issues that make us emulate and seek credibility in the allopathic way, because we will be swallowed up and out-competed by the new conventional medicine that embraces more natural ways.

The tide might seem overwhelmingly against the true essence of the profession. Does that mean we should give up and let naturopathic medicine drift in a direction away from its essence? No. It means that through strength of numbers, with help and support from the CNME, and being true to the medicine in our colleges, clinics, and in practice, the profession will come closer and closer to fulfilling its purpose to humanity. With enough people practicing whole person naturopathy and being effective in the field, we will be able to dispel many of the fears that need not exist in our profession, like the fear of malpractice, the need to be doctors who know everything, and the ominous nocebo effect that surrounds diagnosis and prognosis. In making the changes in our curriculum to accommodate whole person naturopathy courses, we can also dispel the fear of compromising the first principle of our philosophy, "First of all, do no harm." When students have healed themselves, learned to embody love in their practice, and work with the gentle modalities in harmony with the healing power of nature, they become the safest physicians on earth. And when people see naturopaths and remember that being themselves is the most divine and healthy place to be, the worry of appearing unprofessional and flaky will dissipate.

The greatest change that can happen in any educational establishment comes from the students. It is the students actively immersed in the program who recognize what needs to be healed. It is their vigor that pushes for the alignment of all parts of the education with the true vision of our profession. This book, therefore, is a call for all naturopathic students to embrace the philosophy of our medicine and carry it forward in all facets of life. It is a reminder that you are not crazy for believing in the healing paradigm, even if you forget a little going through the grind of the program. Most importantly, it is a call for you to be strong and true—to encourage and celebrate everything in the program that makes you into whole NDs and to topple everything that does not. Do not let any rational arguments of evidence-based thinking make you question yourself. Know that you can tap into the healing power of Nature, the most powerful healing energy that exists. Do not be distracted from the vision of your medicine. Embrace it, be proud of it and watch yourself turn into a doctor of Nature.

What this book is calling you to do, students, administration, and whole NDs, is to cause a revolution until the evolution of naturopathic medicine carries us all back onto our true feet. Rooted in our philosophy, we will continue to establish holism as the foundation in medicine and we will pioneer new discoveries of healing principles for future generations of students and for all of humanity.

Bibliography

Light Emerging: A Journey of Personal Healing, Barbara Ann Brennan, Bantam New Age Books, 1993.

Tao Te Ching, Lao Tse, translation by D.C. Lau, Alfred A. Knopf Inc., 1994.

The Medical Mafia: How to get out of it alive and take back our health and wealth, Guylaine Lanctot, M.D., Here's The Key, 1995.

The Memory of Water: Homeopathy and the Battle of Ideas in the New Science, Michel Schiffe, Harper Collins, 1995.

The Only Planet of Choice: Essential Briefings from Deep Space, 2nd Edition, Transceiver Phyllis V. Schlemmer, Gateway Books, 1996.

Vibrational Medicine: New Choices for Healing Ourselves, Richard Gerber, M.D., Bear and Co., 1988. *Goethe's Way of Science.* State University of New York Press; Albany, NY: 1998. Seamon, D and Zajonc, A; editors

Lindlahr, H, *Philosophy of Natural Therapeutics.* C.W. Daniel Company Limited; Saffron Walden, Essex, England: 1975

Lust, Benedict, *The Naturopathic and Herald of Health*, January 1902, NY.